Advances in Nanomedicine: Nanofibres in Drug Delivery

Advances in Nanomedicine: Nanofibres in Drug Delivery

Michael Mason

AMERICAN
MEDICAL PUBLISHERS
www.americanmedicalpublishers.com

AMERICAN
MEDICAL PUBLISHERS
www.americanmedicalpublishers.com

Cataloging-in-Publication Data

Advances in nanomedicine : nanofibres in drug delivery / Michael Mason.
p. cm.
Includes bibliographical references and index.
ISBN 978-1-63927-554-0
1. Drug delivery devices. 2. Nanomedicine. 3. Nanofibers. I. Mason, Michael.
RS210 .A38 2022
615.19--dc23

American Medical Publishers,
41 Flatbush Avenue,
1st Floor, New York,
NY 11217, USA

ISBN 978-1-63927-554-0 (Hardback)

Contents

Preface

Nanofibres are fibres that measure a billionth of a metre. They have different properties and applications since they are generated from different polymers. Nanomedicine is a branch of medicine that applies nanotechnology to the field of medicine. The applications range from preventing diseases to imaging, diagnosing, monitoring, treating, and regenerating biological systems. The usage of nanofibres in drug delivery significantly lowers the overall drug consumption and reduces the side-effects, and thereby decreases the treatment expenses. This book elucidates the concepts and innovative models around prospective developments with respect to nanomedicine. The various advancements in drug delivery using nanotechnology are glanced at and their applications as well as ramifications are looked at in detail. Scientists and students actively engaged in this field will find this book full of crucial and unexplored concepts.

Various studies have approached the subject by analyzing it with a single perspective, but the present book provides diverse methodologies and techniques to address this field. This book contains theories and applications needed for understanding the subject from different perspectives. The aim is to keep the readers informed about the progresses in the field; therefore, the contributions were carefully examined to compile novel researches by specialists from across the globe.

Indeed, the job of the editor is the most crucial and challenging in compiling all chapters into a single book. In the end, I would extend my sincere thanks to the chapter authors for their profound work. I am also thankful for the support provided by my family and colleagues during the compilation of this book.

Editor

1

Introduction

1.1 Preamble

This volume concerns the potential of drug-loaded polymer nanofibres in pharmaceutics. It is designed to act as a primer for those about to start research in this area, be they new MSc or PhD students or more experienced researchers looking to move into the field. It places significant emphasis on the experimental aspects of fibre production, and provides hints and tips based on the authors' experience throughout to guide readers as they initiate their own experiments. The book can be read as a whole to give a detailed background on pharmaceutical nanofibres, with both experimental insight and an in-depth survey of the key results to emerge from the significant body of literature in this area. Alternatively, it may act as a reference volume to be consulted when embarking on a new series of experiments.

We will begin in this chapter with a brief introduction to the key concepts in pharmaceutical science with which the reader is likely to need to be familiar, including key notions in drug delivery and methods of materials characterisation. In subsequent chapters we will discuss the methods by which nanofibres can be produced, and review some of the most exciting results from this field of research.

1.2 Nanofibres

The convention generally adopted in the literature is that a *nanofibre* is one which has a diameter of below 1 μm, though definitions can vary between disciplines. For example, a broader definition is adopted in industry and engineering disciplines, and submicron fibres are often

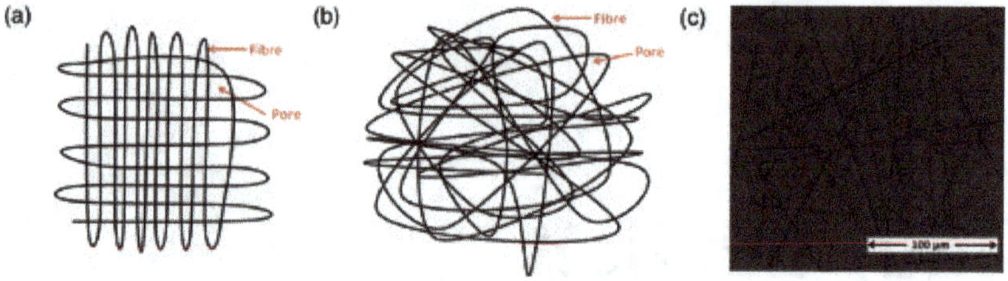

Figure 1.1 Schematic illustrations of (a) woven and (b) non-woven fibre mats, with (c) a microscope image showing a real-life mat (with thanks to Benjamin Yik for the image).

called nanofibres, whereas a stricter definition is employed in biology, and a nanofibre more frequently refers to a fibre with diameter below 100 nm.[1] Depending on their lengths, fibres are categorised as continuous or discontinuous/short fibres, where continuous fibres are defined as having an aspect ratio (length divided by diameter) above 200.

A collection of nanofibres is often referred to as a *mat* or a *mesh*. A mat is termed as either *woven* or *non-woven*, where the former consists of fibres oriented in highly regular patterns, and the latter is randomly orientated. Conventional electrospinning creates a non-woven mat made of a continuous fibre.[2] Schematic illustrations of fibre mats are given in Figure 1.1, together with a microscope image of a real fibre mat.

Continuous nanofibrous mats have very high surface-area-to-volume ratios and offer the advantage of very high porosity, typically ranging between 50% and 99%. By controlling the spinning process, systems with a wide range of fibre size and porosity characteristics can be produced, yielding materials with multiple functionalities. Fibres can be prepared as monolithic systems, where the fibre composition is the same throughout, as core/shell systems with different interior and exterior compartments, or with more exotic multi-component architectures. These properties have caused them to be much explored in the drug delivery setting, as will be discussed subsequently in this volume. Fibres can be prepared from a wide variety of materials, but in the drug delivery context they typically comprise a filament-forming polymer carrier loaded with a drug.

1.3 Key concepts in drug delivery

1.3.1 The therapeutic window and bioavailability

In order to be effective, a drug must be delivered to the right part of the body, at the correct time, and in an appropriate amount. If any one of

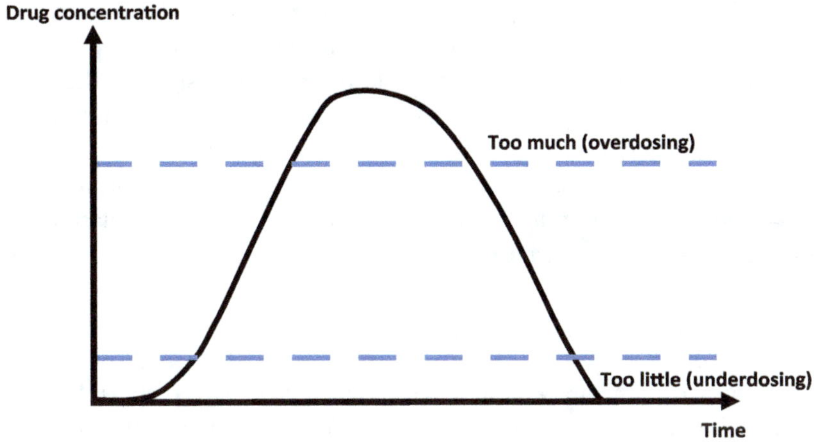

Figure 1.2 An illustration of the therapeutic window. The lower dashed line indicates the minimum plasma concentration required to be therapeutically effective, and the upper line the concentration above which side effects are likely to be experienced. The red line indicates the change in concentration observed with a traditional formulation.

these three criteria is not met, then the medicine will be ineffective or even dangerous. Very frequently, we require the drug to enter the systemic circulation (the bloodstream) for onward transport to its site of action. It is helpful to consider the concept of the *therapeutic window* (Figure 1.2) to understand the issues here.

If the drug concentration is below the bottom line in Figure 1.2, then insufficient drug is present in the bloodstream to relieve symptoms effectively and treat the disease (underdosing). If the drug concentration rises above the upper line, then there is an excess of drug present and (potentially dangerous) side effects can arise; this is known as overdosing. The aim in drug delivery is to maintain the drug concentration between these limits (the *therapeutic window*) to ensure effective yet safe treatment of the patient.

The change in concentration with time which arises with a traditional tablet or capsule formulation is also illustrated in Figure 1.2. The drug concentration rapidly increases to bring the concentration into the therapeutic window, but then the concentration continues to rise until overdosing occurs. The concentration next declines back into the safe region, before dropping below the lower limit of the window. Another dose of medicine will be required at this point in order for the patient to feel continuing relief of symptoms.

At this point, it is helpful to introduce the concept of *bioavailability*. This is a measure of how much of an administered drug reaches the systemic circulation. If a drug is administered intravenously (IV), then the bioavailability is by definition 100%. The absolute bioavailability for a formulation given via another route will be less, and is described relative to the IV value (that is, bioavailability of the drug from formulation $x = 100 \times$ amount of drug in systemic circulation with formulation x / amount of drug in systemic circulation if drug is given IV).

1.3.2 Modified-release systems

The most convenient way to administer a medicine to a patient is through the oral route. Patients are familiar with taking medicines by mouth: this delivery route thus leads to high levels of compliance with the dosage regimen, and is preferred unless there are particular reasons why it is not suitable (e.g. when local delivery is required). More than 70% of medicines are given orally. The majority of these are *conventional* or *immediate-release* dosage forms: such formulations rapidly release the drug in the stomach to provide a swift onset of action. This can be very beneficial when, for instance, the patient is suffering from pain and requires fast alleviation of symptoms. However, in other circumstances such rapid drug release is inappropriate, and other release modalities are required. For instance, for the treatment of maladies lasting longer than a few hours multiple doses will be required using immediate-release formulations.

It is often more desirable to maintain the concentration in the therapeutic window over a prolonged period of time (e.g. 24 h, such that only one dose a day is required), thereby facilitating patient compliance. The term *modified-release* (MR) is used to describe formulations which seek to release the active pharmaceutical ingredient (API) at a particular rate, at particular time points, or to specified sites in the gastrointestinal tract. The major types of MR dosage form are those which are *delayed-release* (which do not release the drug immediately upon application, but rather at some later point in time), *extended-release* (which maintain the plasma concentrations of the API over a prolonged period of time to permit longer intervals between dosing) and *gastro-resistant* (precluding drug release in the stomach, and instead targeting it to a later stage of the gastrointestinal (GI) tract when a particular pH level is met).

MR dosage forms have a number of benefits. Extended-release formulations maintain the plasma drug concentration in the therapeutic window for much longer than immediate-release preparations, including overnight when the patient will not be awake to take multiple doses.

Further, extended- and delayed-release systems can permit APIs to be released when required to match the body's natural circadian rhythms (for instance, diseases such as arthritis are worse in the morning). Side effects can be reduced: in immediate-release formulations, the maximum plasma concentration tends to spike above the upper limit of the therapeutic window, leading to adverse side effects. MR systems ameliorate this problem, reducing the maximum concentration to ensure it lies within the therapeutic window. Reducing the dosing frequency to, for instance, once daily will usually improve patient compliance as the regimen becomes more convenient for the user. Treatment can also be localised to particular regions of the GI tract, which can be required for conditions such as inflammatory bowel disease.

Modified-release systems can be classified conveniently into *reservoir* and *matrix* systems. In a reservoir system, the drug content is surrounded by a membrane which controls the rate of release. In a matrix system, the drug is dispersed evenly throughout a (typically polymer) matrix. This is illustrated in Figure 1.3. These systems can be:

- diffusion-controlled, where the rate of release is determined by how rapidly the drug molecules can diffuse through the rate-controlling membrane or the polymer matrix;
- dissolution-controlled, where the release rate is governed by the speed at which the polymer membrane or matrix dissolves;
- erosion-controlled, where the polymer is not soluble in physiological media but instead is gradually worn away to free the drug loading.

MR dosage forms are often expensive to develop, but they add to the spectrum of treatment options available to healthcare professionals

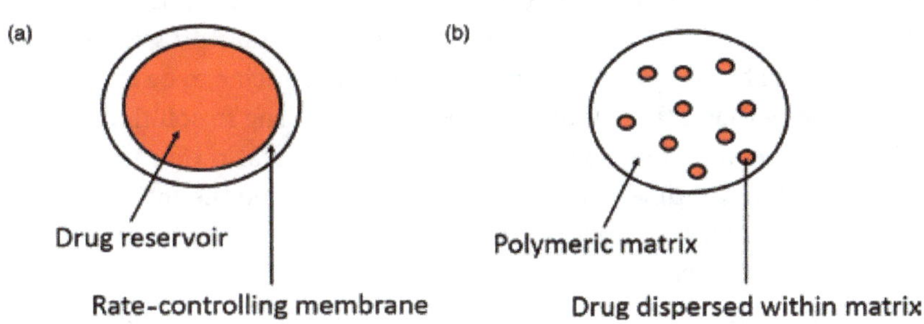

Figure 1.3 Schematic illustrations of (a) reservoir and (b) matrix systems.

and can allow a company to continue to profit from an old and out-of-patent API. They can additionally reduce costs for healthcare systems by improving the quality of disease management. Nanofibres have been used to develop a range of MR formulations, which will be discussed in subsequent chapters.

1.3.3 Dissolution, solubility and permeability

Most frequently, oral formulations are administered in the form of solid materials (e.g. as tablets or capsules). These are convenient for the patient, resulting in typically high compliance with the dosage regimen. Industry also has a wealth of experience in their design, preparation and testing. However, in order to be effective a drug needs to be in solution (individual drug molecules dispersed throughout a liquid solvent): a solid formulation must thus dissolve into solution to be effective *in vivo*. This requires the drug molecules in the solid form to be prised apart, overcoming any intermolecular forces between them, and mixed with the solvent. The strength of the forces between the drug molecules in the solid state will thus help to determine how easy this transition is.

Since physiological fluids comprise mostly water, we require the drug to be water-soluble. Once in solution, however, in the majority of cases the drug then needs to pass through lipid-based biological membranes to reach the systemic circulation. The ability of a drug to achieve the latter is known as its *permeability*.

When considering the dissolution process, two concepts are important: the *solubility* and the *dissolution rate*. Solubility is a capacity term: it refers to the maximum concentration of drug in solution when a solid drug/solvent mixture has been allowed to reach equilibrium. Dissolution rate is a kinetic term, and details how quickly the drug dissolves into solution. The two are distinct but related – it is usual for a highly soluble drug to dissolve quickly, and an insoluble drug to dissolve slowly – and both need to be considered. For a medicine to be effective it is necessary that a therapeutic concentration of drug in solution can be obtained (i.e. a certain solubility is required), and also that the dissolution happens on timescales appropriate for the time the medicine will spend in the digestive tract (so the dissolution rate must also be greater than a certain value).

The permeability/solubility properties of an API are conveniently summarised using the Biopharmaceutical Classification System (BCS; Table 1.1).

Table 1.1 The Biopharmaceutical Classification System

Class	*Solubility*	*Permeability*
I	High	High
II	Low	High
III	High	Low
IV	Low	Low

Class I drugs, with high solubility and high permeability, can be formulated into medicines relatively easily. Class II drugs require careful formulation in order to get them into solution, but once in solution will permeate easily. Class III drugs dissolve easily, but permeation enhancers are required to permit them to pass to the systemic circulation. Class IV drugs are extremely challenging to convert into medicines, since challenges in both solubility and permeability must be overcome. Approximately 35% of drugs on the market fall in class I, with 30%, 25% and 10% in classes II, III and IV, respectively. Increasingly, however, new drug entities fall into classes II, III or IV, leading to numerous challenges in their formulation.

1.3.4 Physical form

Most APIs, in the solid state, are *crystalline materials*. This means that the solid form contains a regular, repeating arrangement of drug molecules extending in three dimensions. The simplest unit or 'building block' of the structure is known as the *unit cell*. If more than one arrangement of molecules is possible in the solid state, then the different arrangements are referred to as *polymorphs*. This is illustrated schematically in Figure 1.4. Different polymorphs will have different unit cells, and because the molecules are arranged differently in the varied polymorphs the intermolecular forces between them (hydrogen bonding, van der Waals interactions, etc.) are also different. This results in different polymorphs having different solubilities and dissolution rates.

Solid-state phases are also possible, in which there are regular arrangements of more than one molecule (or ion) (Figure 1.4). In the pharmaceutical setting, this leads to *pseudopolymorphs*. These contain both the API and a second component in the unit cell. If the API is ionised then a charge-balancing counterion will be present, and we term such phases *salts*. Alternatively, it might be that there is a stoichiometric amount of water (a *hydrate*) or another solvent (a *solvate*) present in the

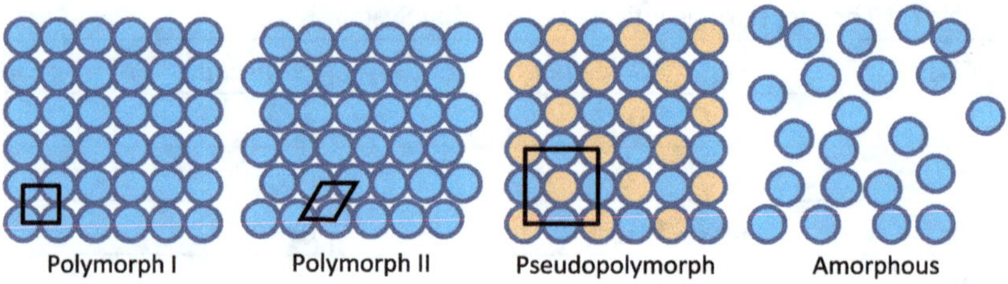

Figure 1.4 Schematic diagrams of two polymorphic forms of an active pharmaceutical ingredient, a pseudopolymorph and the amorphous form. The unit cell is marked in red where applicable.

unit cell. With hydrates and solvates, the co-former is a liquid at room temperature and pressure. If the co-former is a solid at room temperature and pressure, the material is known as a *co-crystal*. Introducing the second component into the solid state causes the intermolecular interactions present to change, and thus pseudopolymorphs will have different solubilities and dissolution rates to crystals of the pure API. As a result, by changing the physical form of the drug, we can alter the *in vivo* performance.

Both for polymorphs and pseudopolymorphs, as well as the arrangement of species in the solid state (the intrinsic properties), it is also necessary to consider the *particle size* and *crystal habit*. Dissolution rate is directly related to the surface area (the larger the surface area, the more rapid dissolution will be) and hence is inversely correlated to particle size (via the Noyes–Whitney equation). Thus, reducing the particle size of a drug should increase dissolution rate and improve bioavailability. Further, the equilibrium solubility of a particle is also inversely related to its particle size (through the Ostwald–Freundlich equation), although this effect is only significant for particles less than 1 μm in size. The crystal habit refers to the particle shape, which can again influence dissolution rate because some faces (sides) of a crystal will dissolve more quickly than others.

The presence of intermolecular forces between molecules in the solid state leads to an energy barrier to dissolution, which must be overcome for the drug to transition from the solid to the solution state. The greater this energy barrier, the lower the solubility and the dissolution rate will be. If the energy barrier could be reduced to zero, then we would expect to see very fast dissolution and very high solubility. This can be achieved by converting the API into the *amorphous form*. Here, the drug molecules are arranged in a random manner in the solid state, and there is no long-range order (Figure 1.4).

(a)

(b)

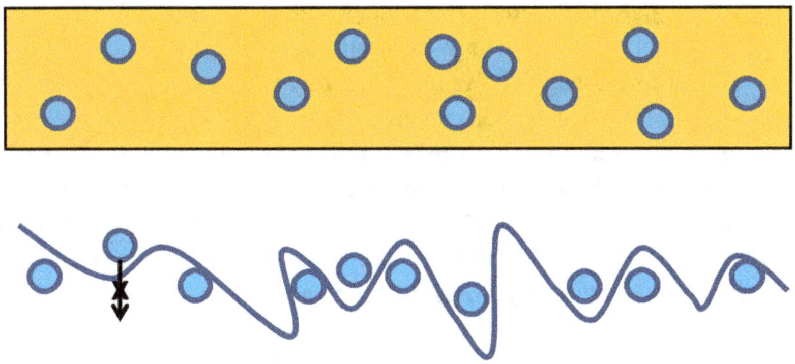

Figure 1.5 (a) A schematic of an amorphous solid dispersion showing the polymer matrix in orange and the drug molecules in blue and (b) an illustration of how the polymer chains block movement of the drug molecules and thus stabilise the amorphous form.

The amorphous form can be very attractive to pharmaceutical scientists, but there is a problem: it is inherently thermodynamically unstable, and thus over time the amorphous form will 'relax' to give a crystalline material. Thus, great care must be taken when making such formulations to ensure that the medicine taken by the patient has the same physical form as that produced in the factory. One way to do this is to blend the drug with a polymer in an *amorphous solid dispersion* (ASD), as illustrated in Figure 1.5. This can stabilise the amorphous form because the polymer provides steric hindrance to the translational movement and reorientation of molecules which are required to transform to the crystalline phase. Polymer-based nanofibres have been used extensively to generate such ASDs.

1.4 Nanofibre characterisation

1.4.1 Electron microscopy

Microscopy allows us to magnify a sample and to inspect features which are invisible to the naked eye. While traditional light microscopy can be of use in the preliminary characterisation of nanofibres, allowing us to confirm the successful formation of fibres (or not), their nanoscale diameters (particularly when below 200 nm) mean that a detailed inspection of the surface morphology or diameter quantification is not possible using this technique. A typical light microscopy image of some fibres of diameter *ca.* 1 μm is given in Figure 1.1(c). The presence of fibres is clear, but even with these relatively large fibres their surfaces cannot clearly be resolved.

Light microscopy allows us to magnify samples by up to 1000-fold (but 100-fold is much more common); to gain more insight, electron microscopy is required. This permits magnification of 100,000-fold to 200,000-fold and nm-scale resolution. Both scanning and transition electron microscopy (SEM and TEM) are used in nanofibre characterisation, with the former being employed to study the fibre surfaces and the latter the interior structure. SEM uses the reflectance of an electron beam from the sample, and requires the sample under investigation to have a conductive surface. This is achieved for polymer fibres by coating them with a thin layer (5–20 nm) of metal, typically gold. SEM allows us to study thicker samples than TEM, since for the latter the electrons need to pass through the sample. However, only with TEM can we explore the interior structure of the materials. Typical SEM and TEM images of nanofibres are shown in Figure 1.6.

1.4.2 X-ray diffraction

X-ray diffraction (XRD) is a widely used technique in solid-state materials characterisation. It relies on the diffraction of a beam of X-rays by a

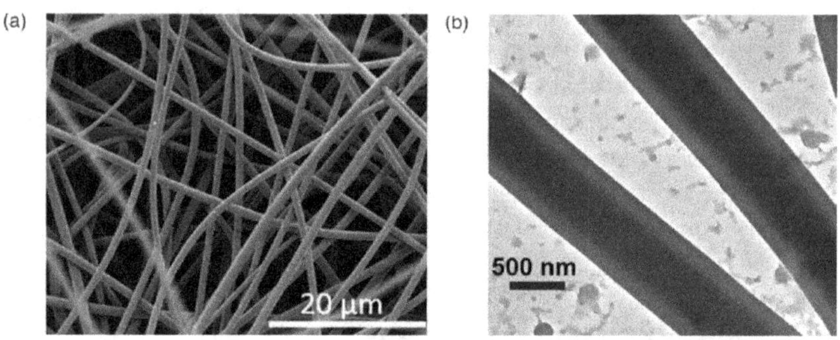

Figure 1.6 Sample (a) scanning electron microscopy (SEM) and (b) transmission electron microscopy (TEM) images of nanofibres. The SEM image provides a clear visualisation of the sample surface, and permits a large area of the sample to be imaged. In contrast, the TEM image considers a much smaller area but allows the interior structure of the fibres to be elucidated. (Reprinted with permission from Illangakoon, U. E.; Yu, D. G.; Ahmad, B. S.; Chatterton, N. P.; Williams, G. R. '5-Fluorouracil loaded Eudragit fibers prepared by electrospinning.' *Int. J. Pharm.* 495 (2015): 895–902. Copyright Elsevier 2015.)

regularly arranged lattice array of atoms or molecules. Because the distance between atoms or molecules in the solid state is comparable to the wavelength of an X-ray, the particular manner in which the components are arranged will lead to a distinct series of diffraction peaks (we term these Bragg reflections). These form an XRD *pattern*, a plot of intensity vs. diffraction angle (2θ). Thus, a crystalline material will have a particular diffraction pattern which can be used as a diagnostic tool to identify it. Different APIs will have different patterns, as will different polymorphs or pseudopolymorphs of a given drug, and through XRD all of these physical forms can be identified.

We can also use XRD to quantify the amounts of phases present in a mixture, and to identify the amorphous form (since there is no regular arrangement of atoms or molecules here, there is no diffraction and no reflections are observed in the pattern). Some exemplar diffraction patterns are depicted in Figure 1.7. In the context of nanofibre drug delivery systems, we employ XRD to determine the physical form of the API in the formulation (most commonly, to discern if it is crystalline or amorphous).

1.4.3 Thermal methods

Differential scanning calorimetry (DSC) is a method by which we can determine the temperature at which a transition happens and the energy associated with it. A sample is loaded into a small metal container (the *pan*), heated at a particular rate and the energy flow is measured during heating. The technique uses a sample pan and a reference pan (which is empty), and both are heated under the same conditions. The amount of energy (heat flow) required to heat the pan loaded with the sample

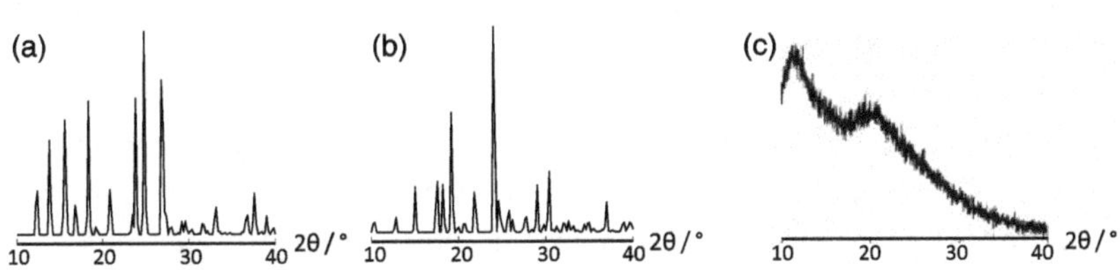

Figure 1.7 X-ray diffraction patterns of (a) paracetamol polymorph I, (b) paracetamol polymorph II and (c) an amorphous material. From a simple comparison of the patterns in (a) and (b) with the literature, it is easy to determine which form is present. Similarly, the amorphous form can easily be identified from its 'halo' appearance and the lack of distinct Bragg reflections.

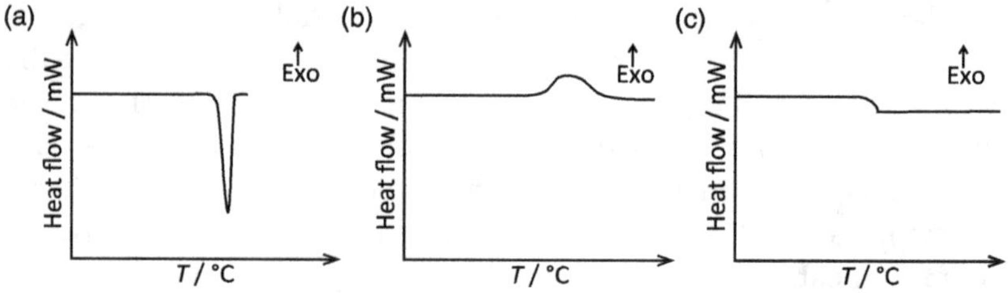

Figure 1.8 Schematic differential scanning calorimetry traces showing (a) melting, (b) recrystallisation and (c) a glass transition. 'Exo' denotes the exothermic direction (heat being given out by the sample).

is compared with the reference pan. Phase transitions such as melting (where a solid material is liquefied) and recrystallisation (the formation of a solid from a molten material) can easily be visualised. This is because, when an API melts, heat must be supplied to break the intermolecular bonds between the drug molecules. This is termed an endothermic transition, and requires the DSC instrument to apply extra energy both to heat the sample and break these bonds. Similarly, if a substance crystallises, intermolecular bonds are formed, and thus energy is given out. These events are manifested as signals in the DSC trace, as illustrated in Figure 1.8.

When working with amorphous systems, there exists another very important event which can be detected by DSC: the glass transition temperature (T_g). This is the temperature at which an amorphous material changes from being brittle to being rubber-like, and is manifested as a change in the baseline of the DSC thermogram (Figure 1.8(c)). Below the T_g, a polymer has low molecular mobility and thus is very brittle and easy to snap. Above T_g, molecular mobility is much higher, and so the material is rubbery and flexible.

DSC is widely used in the characterisation of drug-loaded nanofibres because it allows us to determine what physical form the drug takes (crystalline or amorphous; if crystalline, which polymorph or pseudopolymorph?). We can also use it to observe the presence of water or other solvents in the formulations. If water is present in a hydrate (i.e. there is water inside the unit cell of the crystalline structure), then we will usually see an endotherm at around 100°C followed by an exotherm. These events arise because energy needs to be put into the material to drive away the water, and then the drug molecules will rearrange themselves to form an anhydrous crystal, giving out energy when intermolecular bonds are formed. If water is simply absorbed to the surface or adsorbed inside the body of the fibres, then a broad endotherm will be visible below 100°C, with no subsequent exotherm. Similar considerations apply to other solvents; for instance, ethanol boils at 78°C and so an ethanolate will usually show an endotherm/exotherm pattern at this temperature, while adsorbed or absorbed ethanol will only lead to an endotherm, which will occur at lower temperatures.

To verify the findings of DSC with regard to solvent inclusion, a widely used technique is thermogravimetric analysis (TGA). This measures the mass of a sample as a function of temperature. If a volatile component such as water or another solvent is present in a formulation it will be evaporated upon heating, leading to mass loss. TGA thus allows the amount of the volatile component to be quantified. The temperature at which this occurs (and the ratio of API:volatile component) can be used to verify whether the solvent is present in the unit cell of the crystal or is merely adsorbed or absorbed. The disadvantage of this technique is that, while weight changes can clearly be seen, it is not always possible to determine what may have caused the change leading to possible misinterpretation of results. The combination of TGA with a mass spectrometer or infrared (IR) spectrometer allows an evolved gas to be analysed and its identity confirmed.

1.4.4 Infrared spectroscopy

When molecules absorb IR radiation, the bonds in them vibrate (bend and stretch). Different types of bonds will require different amounts of energy to vibrate, and so the exact wavelength of IR absorbed to cause these transitions is correlated with the types of bonds present. IR spectroscopy thus provides information on the structure of a molecule, since the presence of, for example, C=O, -OH, or $-NH_2$ groups can be discerned. An IR spectrum is a plot of absorbance or transmittance (the two are related through the Beer–Lambert law, $T = 10^{-A}$) vs. the wavenumber ($1/\lambda$) of radiation absorbed. The typical IR frequencies of commonly encountered groups are summarised in Table 1.2.

For solid-state materials, the vibrations of intermolecular bonds between molecules can also be seen through IR spectroscopy. These are referred to as *phonon vibrations* and occur below 1000 cm^{-1}. Typically the pattern of phonon peaks is too complex to unravel fully. In the context of drug-loaded polymer fibres, IR is most commonly used to provide additional evidence on the physical form of the API in the formulation, and to seek insight into any intermolecular interactions present. If the API is amorphously distributed in the carrier, then there will be no or

Table 1.2 The infrared wavenumbers at which common functional groups are seen

Group	*Wavenumber / cm⁻¹*	*Group*	*Wavenumber / cm⁻¹*
O-H stretch	3500–3200	C=C stretch	1680–1640
N-H stretch	3400–3250	N-H bend	1650–1580
C-H stretch	3330–2850	C-H bend	1470–1450
C≡N stretch	2260–2210	C-N stretch	1335–1020
C≡C stretch	2260–2100	C-O stretch	1320–1000
C=O stretch	1760–1665	C-Cl stretch	850–550

minimal API–API interactions, and thus the phonon vibrations of the raw API will not be visible in the IR spectrum. The formation of hydrogen bonds or other intermolecular interactions will result in the change in position or the disappearance of peaks. For instance, where an API has COOH groups, the characteristic C=O stretches will shift in position as a result of H-bonding.

By way of an example, IR spectra for fibres prepared from poly(vinyl pyrrolidone) (PVP) and indomethacin, together with the chemical structures, are presented in Figure 1.9. The full-length spectrum in Figure 1.9(a) demonstrates that indomethacin has many peaks below 1000 cm^{-1}, a number of which will be due to the phonon vibrations of this crystalline material. PVP, an amorphous polymer, has only a few peaks in this region, and most of the API phonon peaks are clearly absent in the spectrum of the drug/polymer fibres. This indicates that the indomethacin was amorphously distributed in the fibres, a hypothesis which was validated using DSC and XRD.[3] The enlargement of the 1800–1500 cm^{-1} (carboxylate) region in Figure 1.9(b) shows that indomethacin has two peaks in this region, at 1712 and 1689 cm^{-1} arising from the COOH and amide groups (Figure 1.9(c)). PVP has a single band at 1654 cm^{-1} from its C=O group. In the spectrum of the fibres, these various carboxylate peaks have merged into a single band at 1660 cm^{-1}, indicating the existence of intermolecular interactions between the API and polymer.

IR spectroscopy is thus very useful to provide insight into both physical form and intermolecular forces. Molecular modelling approaches, in which computational calculations are used to explore the possibility of interactions between species, can be helpful in confirming the interactions suggested from IR spectroscopy. At this point, we should briefly touch on Raman spectroscopy: this is a technique similar to IR

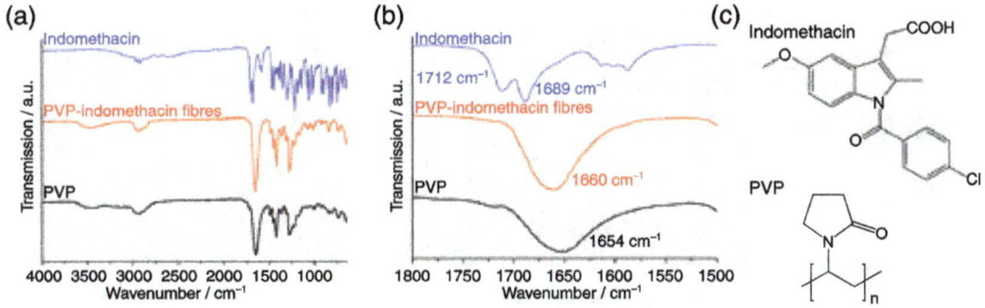

Figure 1.9 Infrared spectra of fibres containing poly(vinyl pyrrolidone) (PVP) and indomethacin, together with chemical structures. The full-length spectra are shown in (a), with an enlarged region in (b) and chemical structures in (c). (Lopez, F. L.; Shearman, G. C.; Gaisford, S.; Williams, G. R. 'Amorphous formulations of indomethacin and griseofulvin prepared by electrospinning.' *Mol. Pharm.* 11 (2014): 4327–4338.)

spectroscopy, but whereas IR spectroscopy uses the absorption of light to generate a spectrum, Raman spectroscopy exploits the scattering of light by vibrating molecules. Both can be used to explore drug-loaded fibres and provide similar information on the stretching and bending of bonds.

1.4.5 Functional performance

1.4.5.1 Dissolution and permeability testing

One of the most crucial attributes of a formulation to be tested is its functional performance. For drug-loaded nanofibres we are typically most interested in the drug release profile, and the amount of drug which can permeate through biological membranes. Exactly how the drug release profile is measured will depend on the application intended: a formulation intended as an oral fast-dissolving system should not be subject to the same release test as one designed for extended release in the small intestine. More details of the precise tests which have been used will be given in subsequent chapters, but one very common assay is *dissolution testing*.

Dissolution, the transition of drug molecules from the solid state into solution, is often the rate-limiting step to drug absorption in the body, and thus an understanding of this can give us an idea of how a formulation will perform *in vivo*. Most often, dissolution testing seeks to mimic the transit of the drug through the GI tract following oral administration.

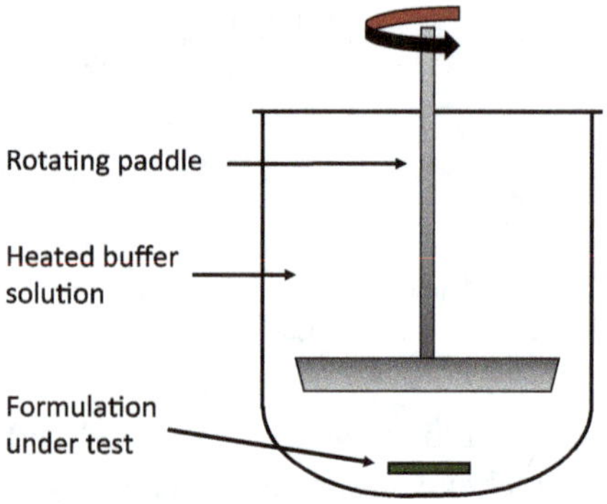

Figure 1.10 A schematic illustration of the US Pharmacopoeia method II dissolution apparatus.

There are well-established tests stipulated in pharmacopoeias which allow for quality control between batches to be maintained, and go some way towards mimicking *in vivo* events. Typically, a formulation is immersed for 2 h in 0.1 M HCl solution (pH 1.0) to simulate the pH of the stomach, and then (if required) in a pH 6.8 phosphate buffer representative of the lower parts of the GI tract. Often this is achieved by starting with 750 mL of the acidic solution and after 2 h adding to that a sodium phosphate solution to raise the pH to 6.8.

The US Pharmacopoeia (USP) lists four different types of dissolution test, of which the most commonly used is probably method II, the paddle method. The apparatus required for this experiment is given in Figure 1.10. In USPII experiments, a formulation is stirred at 50 rpm and 37°C at the required pH. At periodic intervals, an aliquot is removed and the concentration of drug determined using a technique such as ultraviolet (UV) spectroscopy or high-performance liquid chromatography (HPLC). We then construct a plot of percentage release vs. time, which helps us to understand how and where the drug will be released in the body. These tests are not truly representative of what happens in the body – they replace the complex physiology of the GI tract with a litre of a buffer, and do not take into account the precise make-up of the gastric fluids in the body – but because the tests are standardised they permit easy comparison of different formulations. Further, the pharmacopoeias stipulate certain requirements for different dosage forms (e.g. for immediate release, the British Pharmacopoeia states that 80% of the drug should be released within 15 min in the stomach), and dissolution testing allows new materials to be assessed against these standards.

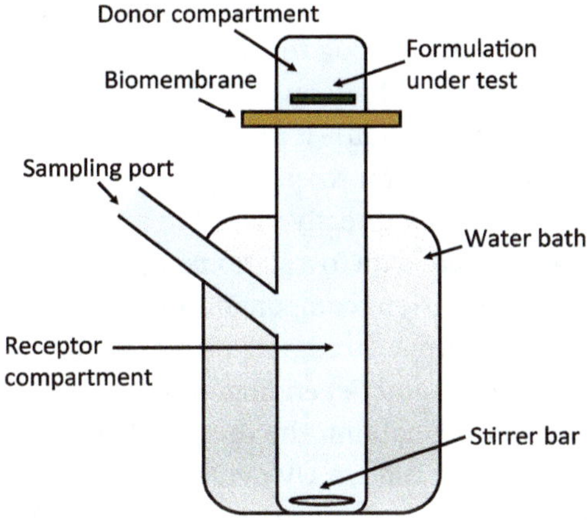

Figure 1.11 A schematic of the typical Franz cell equipment used for permeability testing.

An API, if given orally, must both dissolve into solution from a solid dosage form and also permeate through the biological membranes in the intestine to enter the bloodstream and have systemic activity. Thus, a second commonly performed test is a permeation test. These vary in nature depending on the exact formulation being developed, but all involve investigating the passage of the drug through a biological membrane (or an artificial mimic thereof). Often, porcine intestines are obtained and cut into sections for permeation tests. The formulation is placed in a donor chamber, which is separated from a receptor chamber by the biomembrane; a schematic illustration of this is given in Figure 1.11. A Franz cell is often used for these experiments, but alternative apparatus is also available. Samples are taken periodically from the receptor component to quantify the amount of drug which has passed through the membrane.

1.4.5.2 API quantification

Both the assays described above in section 1.4.5.1 require the amount of API in solution to be quantified. This is achieved using UV-visible spectroscopy or HPLC in the vast majority of cases. UV spectroscopy relies on the fact that APIs usually possess a chromophore (a system of alternating single and double bonds which absorb light in the UV-visible window). The amount of light absorbed is directly proportional to concentration, which means that once a suitable calibration curve has been plotted, UV spectroscopy allows the rapid determination of drug content. Much contemporary dissolution apparatus comes with inline UV monitoring, permitting automated determination of the drug release profile.

In some cases – such as for the simultaneous monitoring of two APIs being released from the same formulation – it can be advantageous to use HPLC. This typically uses a UV detector to quantify the drug concentration, but rather than a sample being directly placed in a UV spectrometer, in HPLC the analyte is first loaded on to a stationary phase (the column), a solid material to which the various components of the sample being analysed will adhere with different strengths. A mobile phase (solvent) is flowed through the column, and depending on the strength of interactions between the API and the column the drug will be freed from the stationary phase at a particular time. A UV detector positioned at the end of the column records the concentration of drug exiting the column as a function of time. HPLC is beneficial because it allows two substances with similar UV spectra to be separated and quantified, and can also lead to more sensitive and accurate detection.

1.4.6 Stability studies

The stability of a formulation is of paramount importance. Inevitably, there will be some degradation of a product upon storage, and it is necessary to understand the rate at which this happens and to set acceptable limits to allow a *shelf-life* to be stipulated. Degradation could take many forms, including chemical degradation of the active ingredient, crystallisation of an amorphous material or microbial contamination. Pharmaceutical scientists often make use of *accelerated ageing studies* to gain rapid insight into these processes and their rates. In such experiments, a formulation is exposed to stress conditions comprising elevated temperatures and relative humidities (RH). These will typically increase the rate at which degradation processes occur – for instance, the amorphous form will convert to a crystalline material more rapidly at 80°C and 80% RH than at room temperature and 50% RH.

The formulation is monitored over a period of time, and the extent of the degradation process at each time is determined using analytical techniques such as those detailed above. This permits the rate of the process to be determined, and the Arrhenius equation ($k = Ae^{-Ea/RT}$) can be used to back-calculate the rate at room temperature, and thus estimate the ultimate shelf-life of the material. This method is far from perfect, because changing the temperature and humidity conditions can change the processes which occur as well as their rates, but it is widely used in the early stages of formulation development to obtain data rapidly. Ultimately the final dosage form will need to be studied under normal storage conditions, but such experiments can take years and are thus not practicable in the early development stages.

1.5 An overview of contemporary pharmaceutical technology

In essence, we can regard the vast majority of drug-loaded fibres as solid polymer/drug composite systems. The simplest way to generate such composites is to use *film casting,* a technique in which a co-dissolving solution of drug and polymer is prepared and the solvent allowed to evaporate to give a film. This is attractive in its simplicity, but suffers from a number of drawbacks in that the process is inherently rather slow (and thus inefficient from an industrial viewpoint) and as a result segregation between drug and polymer can arise. Consequently, researchers have developed a number of alternative methods to accelerate and control the drying process and generate drug/polymer composites from solutions.

At the present time, although drug-loaded nanofibres hold great promise as dosage forms, there are no marketed products based on this technology. It therefore behoves us to consider briefly the most common contemporary pharmaceutical technologies used to prepare polymer/drug composites.

1.5.1 Hot melt extrusion

Hot melt extrusion (HME) has been known as a polymer-processing technique since the early 1930s, and was first explored in the pharmaceutical industry in the 1970s. However, only in the past 20 years or so has it gained significant attention in the drug delivery field. HME has several advantages over traditional pharmaceutical manufacturing processes, including solvent-free processing, rapid fabrication of the final product and the ability to produce formulations able to achieve a wide range of drug delivery patterns.[4] The technique involves heating a mixture of a polymer and API (plus potentially other excipients too) to a point at which it can flow (this could be such that the polymer is heated to above its melting point, T_m, or it may just be heated above its glass transition temperature, T_g). The resultant blend is forced through an aperture under pressure, which both shapes the material and allows intimate mixing between the components. This results in an extended strand of polymer/API blend. Because the extrusion process is continuous it is amenable to scaling up, and the extruded strand can be used as is or undergo secondary processing to give pellets or tablets.

Depending on the polymer used, systems can be prepared which allow for extended release, targeted release, or very rapid release of a poorly soluble active (particularly in the form of an ASD). A number of marketed products are based on HME materials.[5] For instance, Zoladex is an implant based on poly(lactic-co-glycolic acid) produced by AstraZeneca through HME. It contains goserelin acetate as the API, and this is released over up to 90 days for the treatment of prostate cancer. Tablet formulations available include Kaletra (Abbott), a PVP/ poly(vinylalcohol)-based system which releases lopinavir and ritonavir over 6 h for the treatment of human immunodeficiency virus (HIV).

1.5.2 Spray drying

Spray drying is another route widely used to prepare polymer/drug composites. A co-dissolving solution of polymer and API (plus any other excipients desired) is first prepared, and then ejected through an atomiser which generates fine droplets from the bulk solution. The droplets pass into a drying chamber and warm air (or an inert gas) is blown over them. This causes rapid solvent evaporation and results in spherical particles which are recovered in a cyclone unit. The droplets formed during spray drying typically have sizes ranging from less than 10 μm to upwards of 100 μm, which translates to a dry-particle diameter range of 0.5–50 μm.[6] Spray drying is therefore very useful for producing materials for pulmonary administration, where a particle size of 2–5 μm is required for effective delivery to the lung.

Typically, the drug is amorphously distributed in the polymer matrix. By careful control of the inlet temperature, the air flow rate, the humidity of the drying chamber, the type of atomiser and the solution parameters (solvent system, concentration, etc.) it is possible to achieve near-monodispersity in the particle size distribution.[7] Spray-dried excipients are widely used in tablet production, and several marketed medicines also rely on particles produced in this manner. These include Zortress (Novartis; used to prevent organ rejection), Kalydeco (Vertex Pharmaceuticals; indicated for the treatment of cystic fibrosis) and Intelence (Janssen Therapeutics; employed to treat HIV infections).

1.5.3 Freeze drying

Freeze drying (or lyophilisation) is also frequently employed in the pharmaceutical setting. It involves the preparation of a (typically aqueous) solution of drug and polymer, freezing this, and then reducing the pressure such that the water is sublimed to yield a solid drug/excipient composite. The technique is easily scalable, but is rather high-cost and the drying time can be prolonged. Freeze drying is particularly widely used in the preparation of biopharmaceuticals, where maintaining the three-dimensional structure of the active ingredient is both vital and challenging. Medicines such as Synagis (MedImmune; a humanised monoclonal antibody treatment for respiratory syncytial virus) are prepared in this manner, as are some very fast-dissolving formulations such as Nurofen Meltlets (an ibuprofen-containing medicine manufactured by Reckitt Benckiser).

1.5.4 Nanofibre manufacturing

The most common route used to prepare drug-loaded nanofibres is known as electrospinning. This is an electrohydrodynamic (EHD) process in which electrostatic forces are employed to reduce a bulk liquid material down to nanometre dimensions. The details of the process will be discussed in Chapters 2–5, but the basic principles are as follows:

- In the most common process, monoaxial solution electrospinning, a co-dissolving solution of a filament-forming polymer and functional component (API) is prepared in a relatively volatile solvent.
- This is then extruded at a controlled flow rate through a narrow-bore blunt-end metal needle (the spinneret) pointing towards a metal collector, which is usually located at a distance of 10–20 cm.
- A high potential difference (commonly 5–25 kV) is applied between the spinneret and the collector, with the former typically being positively charged and the latter grounded.
- The potential difference causes the polymer solution at the spinneret to stretch rapidly while travelling towards the collector, and generates continuous fibres with diameters typically of the order of nm or µm.

A wide range of modifications can be made to the process to control the morphology and properties of the fibres, and Chapters 3–5 will be devoted to a detailed consideration of these. There also exist other fibre production technologies such as solution blowing, island-sea spinning, melt blowing, centrifugal spinning and electro-centrifugal spinning, which will be discussed in Chapter 6. Several of the processes, including electrospinning, solution blowing and centrifugal spinning, potentially have a number of advantages over more traditional pharmaceutical manufacturing technologies because heat is not required to facilitate solvent evaporation. This can be beneficial in cost terms and allows for easier processing of drugs which are heat-labile. The EHD process is also very rapid, with the solvent evaporating in well under 1 s, which can ameliorate some of the issues encountered with freeze drying (see section 1.5.3).

There are, however, a number of challenges which must be overcome. Electrospinning is known to be scalable, but because it often relies on volatile solvents there are a number of health and safety issues which must be addressed to implement it on an industrial scale. Many of the solvents which work best for electrospinning could have undesirable side effects in humans, and thus great care must be taken to ensure that all the solvent has evaporated during the process. Further, for clinical applications it is vital to ensure that there are very high levels of batch-to-batch consistency, and robust quality control measures must be implemented. We will address some of these challenges in Chapter 7.

1.6 Summary

In this chapter, we have presented a brief overview of the key aspects of pharmaceutical formulation science and technology with which the reader ought to be familiar in order to benefit from the remainder of this book. This has necessarily been a rather superficial treatment, and for more detail we recommend consulting the excellent works detailed in the bibliography below. In the remainder of this volume, we will discuss in more detail the formation of pharmaceutical nanofibres and their use in drug delivery.

Chapter 2 will introduce in detail the fundamentals of the electrospinning technique (the most widely used approach to prepare drug-loaded nanofibres), presenting a discussion of the underlying theory and describing the implementation of electrospinning experiments.

We will then move on to survey the literature to review the most exciting results obtained using electrospun formulations in drug delivery. This will be undertaken starting with the simplest systems, with Chapter 3 considering monolithic fibres (with homogeneous structures throughout), Chapter 4 core/shell materials (with separate inner (core) and outer (shell) compartments), and Chapter 5 Janus fibres (where the two sides of the fibre are different). Chapter 6 is concerned with alternative routes to nano- and microfibre manufacture; it will consider the various approaches available, with examples of the materials which have been prepared using them. Chapter 7 focuses on the next steps for drug-loaded fibres, and will address matters of scale-up and industrial translatability.

1.7 References

1. Kalpakjian, S.; Schmid, S. R., *Manufacturing Engineering and Technology, SI Edition*. 7 ed.; Hong Kong: Pearson, 2013.
2. Reneker, D. H.; Yarin, A. L.; Fong, H.; Koombhongse, S. 'Bending instability of electrically charged liquid jets of polymer solutions in electrospinning.' *J. Appl. Phys.* 87 (2000): 4531–4747.
3. Lopez, F. L.; Shearman, G. C.; Gaisford, S.; Williams, G. R. 'Amorphous formulations of indomethacin and griseofulvin prepared by electrospinning.' *Mol. Pharm.* 11 (2014): 4327–4338.
4. Patil, H.; Tiwari, R. V.; Repka, M. A. 'Hot-melt extrusion: From theory to application in pharmaceutical formulation.' *AAPS PharmSciTech* 17 (2016): 20–42.
5. Tominaga, K.; Langevin, B.; Orton, E. 'Recent innovations in pharmaceutical hot melt extrusion.' www.americanpharmaceuticalreview.com/Featured-Articles/179317-Recent-Innovations-in-Pharmaceutical-Hot-Melt-Extrusion/. Accessed 26 June 2017.
6. Vehring, R. 'Pharmaceutical particle engineering via spray drying.' *Pharm. Res.* 25 (2008): 999–1022.

1.8 Bibliography

Aulton, M. E., Taylor, K. M. G. *Aulton's Pharmaceutics, 5th edition*. London: Elsevier, 2018.

Gaisford, S., Saunders, M. *Essentials of Pharmaceutical Preformulation*. Chichester: John Wiley, 2013.

2

Basics of Electrospinning

2.1 Background

Electrospinning applies a strong electric field (kV range) to disperse liquids into fine jets. For the purposes of this volume, these liquids will comprise polymer solutions, emulsions, suspensions or polymer melts containing one or more active ingredients. Electrospinning, together with electrospraying, are sister electrohydrodynamic (EHD) processes, and both involve charged liquid jets. Depending on the properties of the liquid being handled, the application of electrical energy may yield either fibres (electrospinning) or particles (electrospraying or EHD atomisation). This volume focuses on fibres, and thus most attention will be paid to the former. The difference between the two EHD processes will be discussed in more detail in subsequent sections.

Electrospinning at the laboratory scale is a low-cost route to manufacture near-monodisperse micro-/nanofibres with a high surface-area-to-volume ratio and highly tuneable properties. This lends them to a wealth of applications, including biomedical and healthcare products, photovoltaics and photocatalytic materials, stimuli-responsive and smart robotics, optical and chemical sensors and antimicrobial filters, to list but a few.[1] As a result electrospun fibres have been explored in a broad gamut of research areas – for instance, materials science, life sciences and clinical medicine. Electrospinning is highly versatile and can generate uniform fibres with a large range of diameters. The smallest nanofibres have cross-sections containing fewer than 10 elongated molecules, and the largest diameters can be of hundreds of microns, similar to conventional textile fibres. The porosity of the fibre mat may also be varied over a wide range through systematic changes to the experimental protocol.

In this chapter, we will discuss the key scientific concepts which underpin the electrospinning process, together with the different types of experiment that can be performed and the range of fibres that are produced.

2.2 A brief history of electrospinning

It is only in the last decade or so that researchers have begun to explore the use of electrospun nanofibres in drug delivery, but the EHD process has been studied for centuries. The physical phenomenon underpinning electrospinning was first noted in 1600 by William Gilbert, who described magnetic and electrostatic phenomena in which a droplet could be deformed into a cone shape and a spray of liquid jetted from the droplet when a piece of charged amber was placed close to it. The electric field exerted by the charged amber induced electrostatic charges on the surface of the liquid droplet. When the built-up surface charges overcame the surface tension of the liquid, an aerosol of charged droplets was produced.

Similar observations were made in 1744, when George Mathias Bose reported aerosols produced by applying high electric potentials to liquid droplets at the end of a glass capillary tube. A quantitative explanation emerged towards the end of the nineteenth century: in a series of essays published in 1879 and 1882, Lord Rayleigh calculated the maximum charge that a liquid droplet could carry and remain stable, known as the Rayleigh limit.

Cooley was the first to patent an electrospinning set-up in 1900.[2] This involved the use of auxiliary electrodes to direct fibre deposition on to a continuously rotating reel, similar to the spinning drum in conventional fibre production. Several others have since investigated the phenomenon: in particular, Zeleny's work in 1914–1917 initiated efforts in academia to model mathematically and understand the physics of the EHD process.[3] In the 1930s and 1940s, Formhals registered 11 patents on the process of electrospinning. Many of Formhals' designs laid the foundations for some of the most important contemporary electrospinning set-ups such as needleless spinning,[4] multiple needle set-ups[5] and using parallel electrodes to produce aligned fibres. At the same time, in Russia electrospun fibres were developed into filter materials known as Petryanov filters by Rozenblum and Petryanov-Sokolov. By 1939, the Soviets had commercialised the technology to manufacture electrospun smoke filter elements for gas masks, which found use during the Chernobyl disaster.[6]

Taylor's work during the 1960s provided a mathematical model for the conical shape of the droplet under the influence of an electric field and experimentally confirmed the Rayleigh limit. Taylor's work further underpinned the theoretical understanding of electrospinning, and the conical shape formed at the spinneret during a stable EHD process is often called the Taylor cone.[7]

Furthermore, Simons filed a patent in 1966 describing non-woven patterned fibrous mats collected on metal grids, electrospun from thermoplastics such as polycarbonate and polyurethane.[8] Simons identified key liquid parameters that must be controlled for electrospinning, including solvent properties such as volatility, viscosity, dielectric constant and conductivity. He particularly highlighted the importance of solution viscosity in obtaining continuous fibres.

In addition to solutions, Larrondo and Manley investigated polymer melts as materials for electrospinning. Melt electrospinning is a valuable approach when the polymer, such as many thermoplastics, does not dissolve in common solvents. However, melt spinning is difficult to set up due to the need to maintain a high temperature in the range of 200°C, and the requirement of a higher voltage (above 25 kV) compared to solution electrospinning (below 25 kV in most cases).[9]

Although the aforementioned studies laid the foundation for the electrospinning technique, it was not until the 1990s, with interest in nanoscience and nanotechnology increasing rapidly, that the EHD phenomena enjoyed resurgent attention from researchers, and the name 'electrostatic spinning' gave rise to the now widely used name 'electrospinning'.[10] During this time, work was focused on furthering understanding of the interrelated electrospinning parameters, electrostatics and fluid dynamics under a strong electric field.[11] Since then, the number of publications on electrospinning has seen an exponential increase year on year.

2.3 EHD fundamentals

Electrospinning can be used to process a very wide range of materials, from liquids such as melts to solutions or suspensions of small molecules, biological materials, cells, bacteria and polymers (both natural and synthetic).[12] Here, we are most interested in the electrospinning of polymers, and thus our discussion will centre on the processing of polymers and

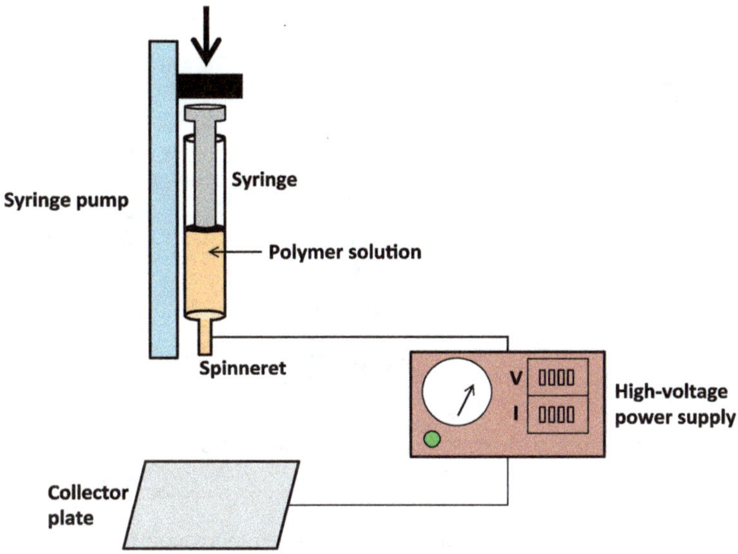

Figure 2.1 A schematic illustration of the apparatus required for electrohydrodynamic experiments.

polymer/drug mixtures. Since the solution approach is more common, the topics will be discussed from this perspective; analogous considerations apply to the processing of emulsions or suspensions.

As explained earlier, electrospinning and electrospraying are 'sister' EHD technologies for the production of polymer-based micro- and nanomaterials. The two are governed by identical theoretical principles and use the same basic equipment. The experimental set-up is illustrated in Figure 2.1.

There are four common components to the basic EHD apparatus: a high-voltage power supply, a precision syringe pump, a syringe fitted with a metal needle (the *spinneret*) and a collector. The power supply is connected to both the spinneret and the collector, with the former usually supplied with either a positive or a negative charge and the latter either grounded or having the opposite polarity to the spinneret. The syringe is filled with a spinnable liquid (e.g. a solution of a polymer, usually with a functional component such as a drug), often referred to as the *working solution*. The solution is extruded through the spinneret at a constant flow rate, controlled by the syringe pump. In conventional electrospinning using a benchtop set-up (described above), a voltage of 5–25 kV is usually applied to the spinneret with a distance of 5–25 cm between the spinneret and the collector. It is worth noting here that, over

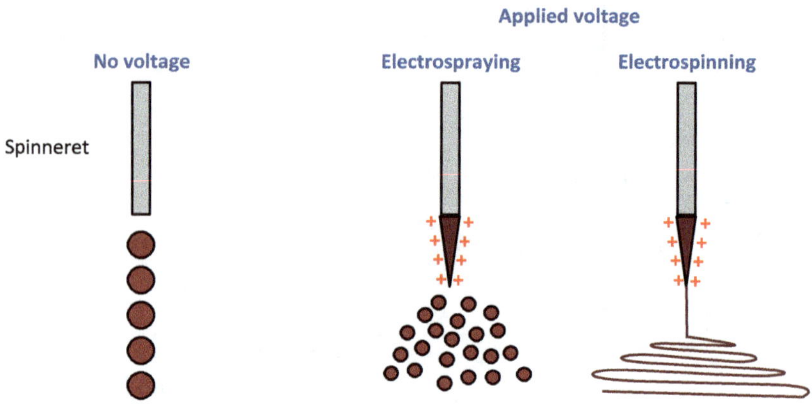

Figure 2.2 A schematic illustration of the formation of the Taylor cone.

the last decade, numerous modifications to the electrospinning apparatus have been reported, allowing direct writing/printing of fibres in precise arrangements. One of the commonly studied variations, near-field electrospinning, can now deposit nanofibres with great precision under a voltage as low as 200 V over a distance of 0.5 mm.[13]

If a solution is dispensed from a capillary with no voltage applied, it will exit in the form of spherical droplets, in order to minimise surface tension (an attractive force which acts to minimise surface area). In electrospinning, when a charge is applied to the spinneret, the solution inside acquires a charge, the magnitude of which is dependent on the applied charge, and the solution conductivity and dielectric constant. Repulsive forces between the charges at the droplet surface and the strong potential difference between the charged solution and the collector cause its spherical shape to deform into a cone shape (the *Taylor cone*; Figures 2.2 and 2.3). In electrospinning, at the tip of the cone the polymer solution emits a jet, which rapidly elongates and reduces in diameter. The jet travels away from the spinneret, with the solvent evaporating as the charged solution moves towards the collector. When the jet reaches the grounded collector it discharges. Typically, by this time the solvent has been exhausted, and thus solid products are obtained. As mentioned in section 2.2, electrospinning is strongly dependent on the physical properties of the polymer solution as well as the processing parameters employed.[14] These will be discussed in more detail in sections 2.4 and 2.5.

When the Taylor cone emits a polymer jet, electrospinning occurs to yield fibre products. However, it is also possible that the cone breaks up into droplets: this is electrospraying (Figure 2.2). Similarly to the

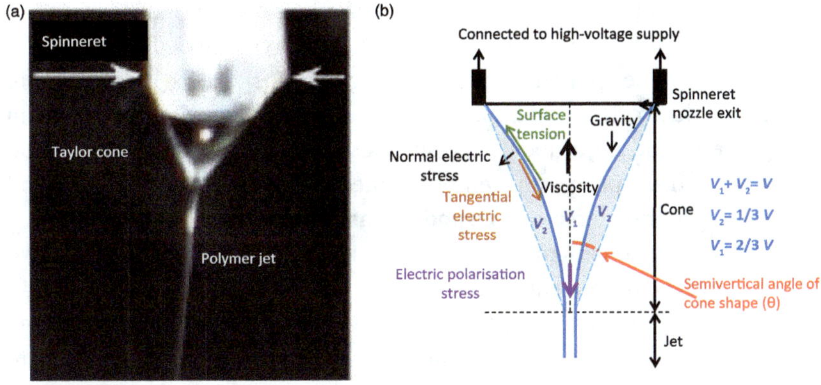

Figure 2.3 (a) A digital photograph of the Taylor cone and ejected polymer jet observed in a typical electrospinning experiment. (Modified with permission from Yu, D.-G.; Williams, G. R.; Gao, L.-D.; Bligh, S. W. A.; Yang, J.-H.; Wang, X. 'Coaxial electrospinning with sodium dodecylbenzene sulfonate solution for high quality polyacrylonitrile nanofibers.' *Colloids Surf. A* 396 (2012): 161–168. Copyright Elsevier 2012.) (b) A geometric diagram of a symmetric liquid cone with a thin jet at its apex, depicting forces acting on the cone jet. V is the volume of the conical frustum (i.e. the shape left when the top part of the cone has been cut off), V_1 is the jet volume and V_2 is the space the jet is not occupying in the conical frustum.

electrospinning process, the droplets lose solvent and shrink as they move towards the collector, typically being deposited on it as spherical particles. The explanation for the difference between spinning and spraying lies in the solution properties and processing parameters.

For both electrospinning and spraying, most reports in the literature apply a positive potential at the spinneret. However, it should be noted that the voltage is not constrained to positive polarity, although negative polarity has been reported to produce fibres with larger average diameter.[15]

2.4 Understanding the electrospinning process

Electrospinning involves a range of interlinked parameters broadly categorised into material (here we focus on solution) parameters and processing parameters. Electrospinning is in many ways similar to conventional fibre spinning in textile production. The jet initiated during fibre spinning is generally subjected to tensile, rheological, gravitational, inertial and aerodynamic forces. The difference between electrospinning and conventional textile spinning lies in the origin of the tensile force initiating the fibre jet. In electrospinning, free charges carried by the liquid interact with the applied electric field and the tensile force inducing fibre jetting is due to the potential difference between the charged liquid in a spinneret and a grounded collector. On the other hand, conventional industrial fibre processing employs mechanical means (spindles and reels) to generate tensile force and initiate fibre formation.

Factors influencing electrospinning include rheology, electrostatics, hydrodynamics and the transport of heat, mass and charge within the polymer jet. For simplicity, electrospinning can be divided into three stages: jet initiation, jet elongation and solidification of the jet to generate fibres. A detailed understanding of the underlying physics is not required for the purposes of this volume, but some insight into the processes underway is useful. For more in-depth discussions, the interested reader is invited to consult recent reviews.[1b, 12, 16]

2.4.1 Jet initiation

The charging of a droplet at the spinneret exit is usually the first step in electrospinning. When a polymer solution is supplied by a syringe pump to the spinneret without an applied voltage, droplets form at the exit and fall off under the influence of gravity. This dripping can continue even with the presence of an applied voltage, and ceases only when the electric field becomes sufficient to balance the surface tension of the liquid.

With the application of voltage, a charge is induced on the surface of the liquid droplet as it exits the spinneret. Repulsions between the like charges in the solution act to oppose the forces of surface tension, causing the droplet to change shape from spherical to conical (Figure 2.3(a)). Taylor supplied a mathematical model for the conical shape of the droplet under the influence of an electric field, showing that a conducting liquid can exist in the form of a cone under the action of an electric field when the semivertical angle θ (Figure 2.3(b)) is approximately 49.3°.[7, 9a] A critical voltage, V_k, is required to transform a spherical droplet to a cone shape at the end of a needle connected to one of the electrodes, and can be predicted based on the semivertical angle using Equation 2.1[7b]:

$$V_k^2 = \frac{4H^2}{L^2}\left(\ln\frac{2L}{R} - 1.5\right)\left(\left(2\cos 49.3^\circ\right)\pi RT\right)\left(0.09\right) \qquad \text{Equation 2.1}$$

In Equation 2.1, H is the spinneret-to-collector distance (in cm), L is the length of the spinneret (cm), R is the inner radius of the spinneret exit (cm) and T is the surface tension of the fluid (dyn cm^{-1}). All these factors will therefore have an effect on the voltage that needs to be applied to initiate the spinning process. Further, the semivertical angle can also vary with different polymer solutions and melts, and hence the critical voltage required to generate the cone shape droplet varies with different electrospun materials.[17]

Following the establishment of a conical-shaped droplet at the spinneret exit with a sufficiently high applied voltage, additional surface area needs to be created by some means to accommodate the charge build-up on the conical surface. This occurs through the formation of a 'cone jet'. The formation of the Taylor cone and ejection of the jet can be clearly seen by eye in electrospinning experiments (Figure 2.3(a)). A geometric model of a stable cone jet is given in Figure 2.3(b), and illustrates the forces at play during an electrospinning cone jet process.

It is important to be aware of the electric field gradient in the electrospinning experiment. The average gradient (V cm^{-1}) is often described as the potential difference divided by the spinneret-to-collector distance. The resultant value is a good approximation of the field near to the collector. However, the electric field close to the tip of a Taylor cone, just before jet emission, is much higher. After the point of jet emission, the electric field varies across the distance between spinneret and collector in a manner dependent on the surrounding environment. That said, in the interests of establishing functioning experimental parameters, the average field gradient is a sensible parameter to consider when deciding on the voltage and spinneret-to-collector distance being used. In order to operate an efficient and reproducible production process, when varying applied voltage during process optimisation one should keep the collection distance constant to ensure meaningful and systematic optimisation of the field strength.

2.4.2 Electrospinning vs. electrospraying

The distinction between electrospinning and electrospraying depends on the stability of the electrified liquid jet, governed by what is known as Rayleigh instability.[18] The latter depends on the molecular entanglements in the liquid (a frequently used analogy is to imagine polymer chains in a solution as snakes slithering over one another).

There are two key forces acting on the surface of the cone jet, and these oppose one another. Electrostatic repulsion of the charges in the solution promotes an increase in surface area to minimise these repulsions. This drives the charged polymer jet emitted from the Taylor cone to become longer and narrower. Acting against this, the surface tension seeks to reduce the total surface area of the jet. Which of the two opposing forces prevails depends on the properties of the fluid being processed, particularly its viscosity and surface tension.

Viscosity is a reflection of the degree of molecular entanglement in the liquid,[19] and is fundamental in determining whether a material can be employed to form fibres or not. In electrospraying, the molecular entanglement of the liquid is insufficient to overcome the Rayleigh instability; thus, surface tension prevails and the electrified jet breaks up into small charged particles to minimise surface area.[11a, 20] Electrostatic repulsions between the charged droplets prevent them from coalescing, and as the solvent evaporates the particles shrink. This causes an increasing charge density at their surfaces, and so they break up into even smaller droplets (hence the name EHD atomisation). Electrospraying arises with low-viscosity solutions (i.e. those which flow easily; water has low viscosity, while honey is a high-viscosity fluid). In electrospinning the viscosity of the liquid is high and the molecular entanglements present are sufficient to overcome Rayleigh instability within the charged cone jet. Therefore, instead of capillary break-up the jet takes the form of a fibril undergoing a rapid whipping motion. The jet will elongate and its diameter will decrease until a dried fibre is deposited on the collector.

The molecular weight of the polymer strongly influences the degree of molecular entanglement of the polymer solution, and is thus very important in ensuring electrospinning rather than electrospraying is performed. The explanation for this lies in the manner in which the molecules in a solution interact. Small molecules can easily flow past one another, giving low-viscosity solutions. In contrast, long-chain polymer molecules are able effectively to become wrapped around one another, leading to entanglement. This is illustrated in Figure 2.4.

As a simple analogy, it can be helpful to think about the difference between cooked rice and noodles. Grains of rice are small and exist as discrete units; it is thus very easy to remove a single grain of rice from a bowl. In contrast, noodles are long and narrow, and when placed in a bowl will become wrapped around one another. Extracting a single noodle from the bowl is rather difficult. The same is true for solutions, and a suitable degree of entanglement is critical for successful electrospinning because the tangling of the polymer molecules helps the jet elongation force to outweigh the surface tension. This ensures that the jet continues to the collector to form solid fibres, and does not break down into droplets. Entanglement can be promoted through the use of

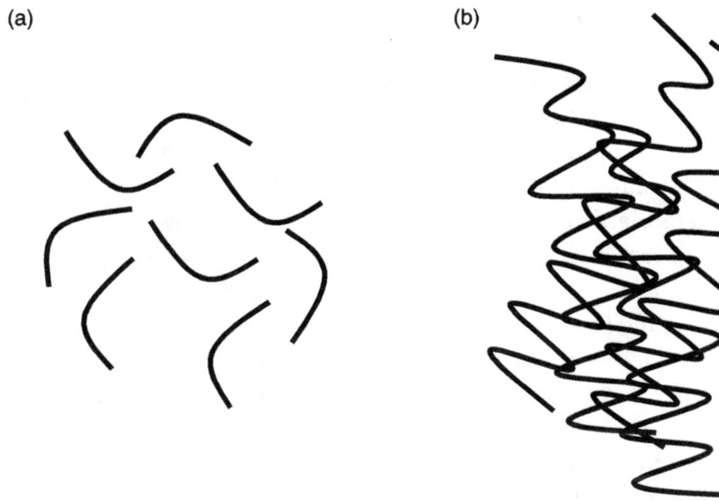

Figure 2.4 The concept of entanglement. (a) Small molecules and low-molecular-weight polymers cannot effectively overlap and entangle. Instead, they flow easily past one another. This leads to low-viscosity solutions which suffer from Rayleigh instability. (b) High-molecular-weight polymers undergo effective entanglement, meaning the force of elongation outweighs the surface tension and permitting electrospinning to be performed.

higher-molecular-weight species and elevated concentrations. However, care must be taken because if the viscosity is too high then spinning will be unstable, resulting in heterogeneous fibre diameters or discontinuous fibres. Moreover, the solvent may deplete quickly at the spinneret exit, leading to blockage.

In addition, it is useful to describe here the 'bead-on-string' or necklace-like morphology of fibres sometimes observed during electrospinning. Bead-on-string arises from a situation intermediate between electrospraying and electrospinning, when charge repulsion and viscous forces are momentarily overcome by the surface tension of the charged liquid. This is often an intermittent occurrence during fibre elongation and considered a defect, resulting in a chain of droplets connected by fibrils. Careful control of the processing parameters during electrospinning can reduce this phenomenon. Methods to avert bead-on-string morphology include moderately increasing the viscosity of the solution either by increasing polymer molecular weight or concentration, or adding surfactants to decrease the surface tension of the solution.

2.4.3 Jet elongation: bending and whipping

As the charged liquid jet travels from the Taylor cone to the collector, it initially follows a linear trajectory (known as the *straight jet*), as it is attracted by the oppositely charged (or grounded) collector. During its journey, it is subjected to a variety of forces with opposing effects. The physical details are out of the scope of this volume and we do not need to consider them in detail here, but the result is that the linear jet does not continue all the way to the collector.[21] Instead, it undergoes what is termed *whipping instability* (also known as bending mode instability or bending instability). This is a rapid elongation process that involves long-waveform perturbations of a liquid column driven by the lateral electric force (Figure 2.3(b)) and aerodynamic interactions, resulting in the jet bending or stretching. This is key in reducing the jet diameter to the nanometre scale to yield nanofibres.

The repulsive Coulombic forces between the charges carried within the polymer solution cause the jet to elongate and narrow continuously until it solidifies. Initially, this results in the emission of a straight jet, but as the jet grows longer the solvent evaporates and the diameter of the jet decreases. The surface charge density of the fibre concomitantly increases, which leads to a further increase in repulsive forces in the jet. Consequently, an increasing amount of time is required to distribute the repulsive charges along the jet length, and therefore it accelerates towards the collector. This produces an extremely high velocity at the leading end of the straight jet. As a result, at a certain point the jet bends and follows spiralling loops (Figure 2.5). Each subsequent loop grows larger in diameter as the jet grows longer and thinner.[1a, 11c] There are repulsions between each segment of the loop, since all parts of the jet bear the same charge, which means the jet follows a bending and whipping pattern before it solidifies on the collector.

The jet may also split into several smaller jets when electrospinning becomes unstable, a phenomenon termed *splaying* or *branching*.[11c] This occurs because of changes in the shape of the jet and/or its charge per unit volume which can arise during the process of jet elongation and loss of solvent. Such changes shift the balance between the repulsive Coulombic forces and surface tension, such that the jet becomes unstable. To reduce the charge per unit surface area, a smaller jet is ejected from the surface of the primary jet. This tends to be seen in highly concentrated and viscous solutions, as well as at very high field strengths.[1a] Splaying should ideally be avoided in the use of electrospinning to produce drug delivery systems, since it leads to inhomogeneities in the products, which can

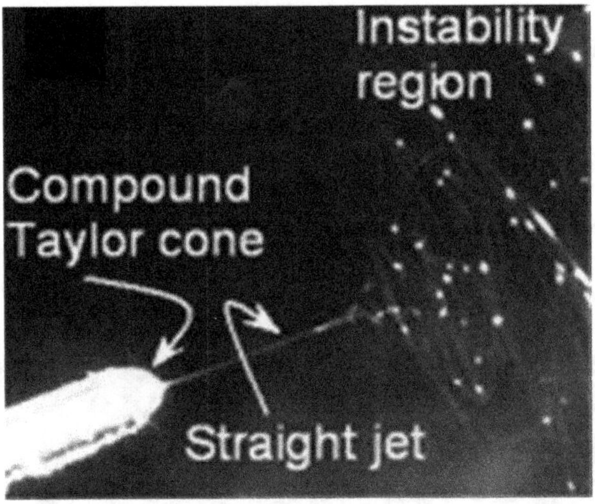

Figure 2.5 A digital photograph depicting bending instabilities during an electrospinning experiment. (Modified with permission from Yu, D. G.; Yu, J. H.; Chen, L.; Williams, G. R.; Wang, X. 'Modified coaxial electrospinning for the preparation of high-quality ketoprofen-loaded cellulose acetate nanofibers.' *Carbohydr. Polym.* 90 (2012): 1016–1023, with permission from Elsevier. Copyright Elsevier 2012.)

preclude the robust and reproducible generation of materials with the desired properties.

2.4.4 Jet solidification

When all the solvent has been exhausted, the jet will become solid. This solidification results in the deposition of dry fibres on the collector.[16] Solvent evaporation begins as soon as the liquid jet is initiated, and increases as the jet undergoes whipping instability. As described in section 1.2, the fibres will collect as a non-woven mesh known as the *fibre mat*. The solidification rate is controlled by the concentration of the solution, the voltage, the spinneret-to-collector distance, the boiling point of the solvent system being used, the environmental temperature and humidity and the surrounding air movement. It is important to balance these to ensure that a dry fibre is produced and the electrospinning process can be undertaken continuously. If solidification happens too quickly (which can occur if the polymer concentration is very high, or the solvent very volatile), then the solution can solidify on the spinneret. This not only results in loss of material but also can block the spinneret.

If the solvent is not all exhausted when the fibres reach the collector then the products are likely to have defects, and not comprise smooth cylindrical fibres. Residual solvent in the fibres may evaporate subsequently, leading to internal voids or porosity being developed and the fibres collapsing in on themselves. This causes their surfaces to wrinkle and/or the fibres to become flattened (Figure 2.6). Alternatively, re-dissolution of the polymer in the solvent may occur, resulting in layers of fibres merging together.

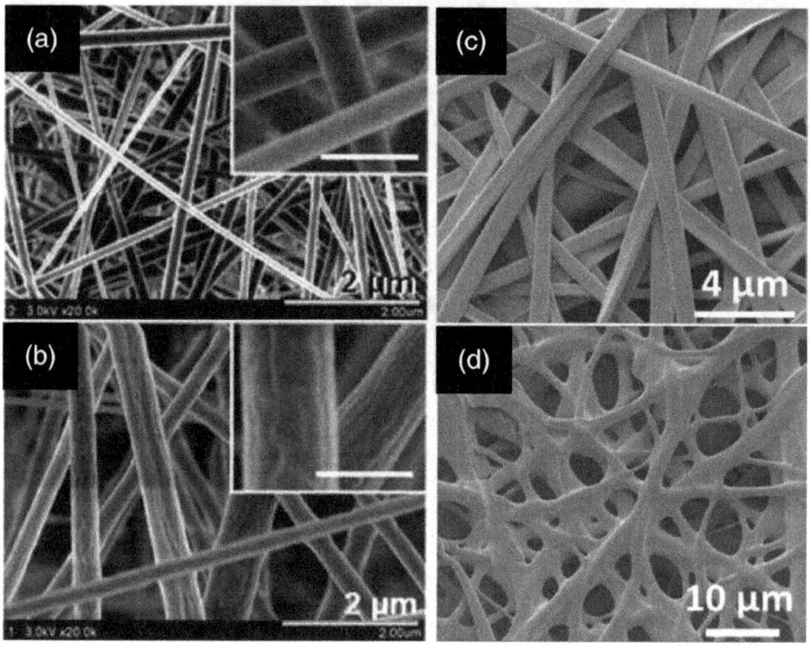

Figure 2.6 Defects that may arise during fibre solidification, showing (a) smooth, cylindrical fibres resulting from a well-optimised process; (b) flattened fibres; (c) wrinkled fibres; and (d) merged fibres. (Images (a) and (b) are modified with permission from Yu, D. G.; Yu, J. H.; Chen, L.; Williams, G. R.; Wang, X. 'Modified coaxial electrospinning for the preparation of high-quality ketoprofen-loaded cellulose acetate nanofibers.' *Carbohydr. Polym.* 90 (2012): 1016–1023, with permission from Elsevier. Copyright Elsevier 2012. Images (c) and (d) are modified with permission from Jia, D.; Gao, Y.; Williams, G. R. 'Core/shell poly(ethylene oxide)/Eudragit fibers for site-specific release.' *Int. J. Pharm.* 523 (2017): 376–385, with permission from Elsevier. Copyright Elsevier 2017.)

During the drying process, *conglutination* can also occur. This is a process by which partially solidified jets come into contact, resulting in fibres that are fused together at these points of contact. The attachments dictate the mechanical properties of the fibre mat, with more contact points making it more rigid.

2.5 The parameters affecting electrospinning

The electrospinning process is affected by many parameters, which can helpfully be divided into solution, processing and environmental parameters. Solution parameters include the polymer molecular weight and structural conformation (these strongly influence the minimum concentration and viscosity required to form continuous fibres) and the choice of solvent or solvent mixtures (which strongly influences surface tension, rate of evaporation, dielectric constant and electrical conductivity). Processing parameters are dependent on the electrospinning apparatus design, but chiefly comprise the applied voltage, spinneret-to-collector distance and the solution flow rate. Each parameter will influence the morphology of the fibres obtained. Through their optimisation and control it is possible to tune the electrospinning process to yield nanofibres with the desired morphology and diameters. In addition, environmental parameters – the humidity, temperature and air circulation speed of the surroundings in which the process takes place – are also important to consider. These are described briefly below, and discussed in more detail in subsequent chapters.

2.5.1 Solution parameters

The fibre formation process relies on the elongational stretching of the polymer solution exiting the spinneret. The dominant influence of the properties of the polymer solution on the electrospinning process and the resultant fibre morphology cannot be overstated. The properties of the polymer solution, such as viscosity, surface tension, conductivity, dielectric constant and volatility, change with the molecular characteristics of the polymer, the concentration of the polymer in solution, and the choice of solvents used. Understanding the polymer solution brings profound insight in achieving a successful electrospinning process.

Key solution parameters which need to be considered are as follows.

Concentration: The concentration of the polymer in solution is a determining factor for the formation as well as diameter and morphology of the fibres from electrospinning. A critical minimum concentration c_e is needed to allow sufficient molecular chain entanglement to overcome surface tension and prevent the electrospinning jet from breaking up. Concentrations below c_e will produce droplets when electrified (electrospraying). At concentrations above c_e, electrospun fibre diameter increases with increasing polymer concentration and the frequency of bead-on-string defects decreases, eventually leading to the formation of beadless uniform nanofibres. The value of c_e is dependent on the molecular chain length, macromolecular structure and the solvent(s) selected to dissolve the polymer.

Molecular weight and molecular chain length: The polymer molecular weight inversely affects the value of c_e required to enable electrospinning.[22] A polymer molecule generally has a long chain-like geometry, but these chains may be branched and there may be crosslinks between chains. These characteristics depend on the polymer's chemical structure and the synthesis method. A linear polymer with a high molecular weight (above 3000 g mol^{-1}, preferably above 10,000 g mol^{-1}, and more preferably above 50,000 g mol^{-1}) leads to a lower c_e for fibre formation in electrospinning than a branched polymer with low molecular weight when dissolved in the same solvent.

Solution viscosity: Viscosity reflects the degree of polymer molecular chain entanglement in a solution. The solution viscosity is influenced both by the molecular weight of the polymer and the properties of the solvent used. Hence, it can be adjusted by both varying polymer concentration in solution and/or changing the solvent. The minimum solution viscosity required to enable electrospinning is that of a solution with polymer concentration higher than the relevant c_e value.

If the viscosity is very low, then electrospraying will occur and the products will comprise particles. An intermediate viscosity will lead to beaded fibres (a situation intermediate between electrospraying and spinning). The effect of viscosity on fibre morphology is depicted schematically in Figure 2.7.

It might therefore be thought that the higher the viscosity the better, but unfortunately the situation is not that simple. A greater viscosity will make it more difficult for the jet to become elongated and narrow, thus leading to thicker fibres. Helix-shaped fibres have also been observed when working with very-high-viscosity solutions,[23] and incomplete drying of a high-viscosity jet can lead to the formation of flattened ribbon-like fibres.[24] Finally, if the viscosity is too high the polymer solution may solidify on the spinneret, leading to it becoming blocked.

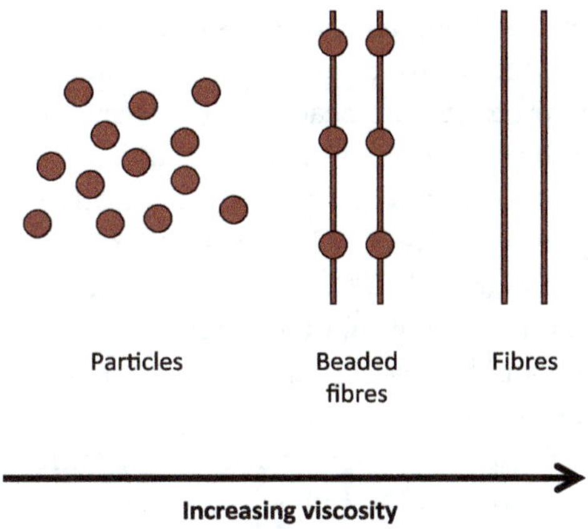

Figure 2.7 The effect of solution viscosity on the products from electrohydrodynamic processing.

The range of viscosities that allows electrospinning is specific to the polymer and solvent system used. For example, Doshi and Reneker found that the optimum viscosity range for electrospinning poly(ethylene oxide) (PEO) nanofibres is 800–4000 mPa s.[21] On the other hand, in a comprehensive investigation on electrospinning poly(acrylonitrile) dissolved in dimethyl formamide (DMF), Baumgarten observed that smooth submicron fibres could be electrospun when the viscosity of the solution was 170–21500 mPa s.[25]

Surface tension: Surface tension acts together with the viscosity of the polymer solution to oppose the electrical drawing force. To begin the electrospinning process, the surface tension must be overcome by the repulsive forces between the charges in the polymer solution. In Equation 2.1, the critical voltage for cone formation V_k is proportional to surface tension T, and thus liquids of higher surface tension require higher V_k for electrostatic processing. However, a higher electric field also means greater potential leakage of the surface charge on the jet into the surrounding air. This makes the cone jet unstable, leading to defects and non-uniformity in the fibres. Defects such as bead-on-string formation can arise when the surface tension of the solution briefly overcomes the elongational forces.

Solutions with very high surface tensions can thus be difficult to spin, as they require significantly stronger electric force to overcome this. In addition, the higher the surface tension, the greater the forces opposing jet elongation, and thus the more likely it is that it will break up into droplets or form bead-on-string defects.

At a fixed polymer concentration, reducing the surface tension has been reported to be an effective route to improve the morphology of the electrospinning product from beaded fibres to smooth fibres.[23] Most solvents used for electrospinning have relatively low to moderate surface tensions (20–45 mN m^{-1} at 20°C), but working with water, a high surface tension solvent (72.75 mN m^{-1} at 20°C) with low volatility (boiling point at 100°C) can be problematic. Surfactants can be added to the working solution to reduce surface tension if required, but these will be carried through into the fibre products, which may be undesirable.

The surface tension of a polymer solution is temperature-dependent, but also varies with the choice of solvent(s), and the concentration and the chemical structure of the polymer. As the electrospinning jet travels towards the collector, solvent evaporation leads to an increasing polymer concentration in the jet. The surface tension of the jet is therefore likely to evolve upon exiting the spinneret and landing on the collector.

Electrical conductivity: The greater the electrical conductivity of the solution, the more easily charge can accumulate in it to build up sufficient tangential stress for fibre elongation, and hence the lower the voltage required to initiate jet electrospinning. Fibres with thinner diameters also result from more conducting solutions. The addition of trace amounts of inorganic salts or ionic organic species to the solution offers a simple route to enhance electrical conductivity, if required. Solutions of zero conductivity cannot be electrospun. However, if the electrical conductivity of the liquid is too high, electrical discharge into the surrounding air will occur, resulting in unstable jetting or halting the electrospinning process altogether. For instance, Morota *et al.* found that increasing the conductivity of aqueous solutions of PEO changed the stable cone jet to an unstable multijet, and solutions with conductivity above 0.5 S m^{-1} could not be electrospun.[26]

Dielectric constant: A temperature-dependent property, the dielectric constant ε (otherwise known as the relative permittivity) of a substance is a measure of the extent to which it concentrates the electrostatic lines of flux when placed in an electric field. It is defined as the ratio of the amount of stored electrical energy when a voltage is applied relative to the permittivity of a vacuum. Solvents of different dielectric constant values interact with the electric field differently during solution electrospinning. Solutions in solvents of an appropriately high range of dielectric constants (ε value above 30 at 20°C) allow a more even distribution of the surface charge on the jet, and have been reported to be easier to electrospin and to produce fibres with smaller diameters.[27]

Volatility: Solvent evaporation has a significant effect on fibre morphology and diameter. Selecting a relatively volatile solvent allows the fibre to dry completely upon reaching the grounded collector, avoiding defects such as fused wet fibres. However, solvent volatility also affects the kinetics of phase separation and hence the morphology of the electrospun fibres obtained. Highly volatile solvents can cause a hard solidified shell to form on the elongating fibre before complete drying can occur, trapping the solvent inside the fibre. As the residue solvent slowly diffuses out of the fibre shell, defects such as wrinkled or porous surface morphologies can occur. In addition, rapid solvent evaporation from the jet can hinder the production of smaller fibre diameters, since there is less time for elongation before complete solidification occurs. Hence, volatile solvents such as acetone, dichloromethane and chloroform are often reported to generate fibres with a larger average diameter than solvents such as water and DMF (though other solvent properties such as water and DMF having moderately high dielectric constants can also contribute to such observations).

Solvent choice: The choice of solvent or solvent mixture strongly influences the viscosity, surface tension, electrical conductivity, dielectric constant and volatility of the solution, and thus is of crucial importance. The selected solvent must not only provide appropriate electrical conductivity, viscosity and surface tension, but also needs to be able to dissolve/disperse the polymer and the functional component of interest at appropriate concentrations.

In general, it is useful to know that using a solvent of lower solubility for the polymer(s) of interest can enhance nanofibre formation or dramatically change the value of the critical concentration, c_e.[28] For example, Shenoy *et al.*[22] found that poly(vinylidene fluoride) (PVDF: molecular weight (Mw) 180 kDa) fibres can be electrospun at concentrations as low as 7.5% w/w using acetone, whereas a concentration of 30% w/w PVDF in DMF was necessary for successful electrospinning. In this case, acetone was a marginal solvent for PVDF whereas DMF was a good solvent. The addition of acetone to the PVDF solution in DMF significantly lowered the c_e necessary for fibre formation.

2.5.2 Processing parameters

Process parameters include the operating parameters (such as applied voltage, flow rate, diameter of the spinneret inner orifice and collection distance), the spinning environment (temperature and humidity) and the set-up design (e.g. the choice of material used as the collection substrate).

Voltage: A sufficient voltage must be applied to initiate jet formation, and as discussed above, this threshold voltage depends mainly on solution properties such as surface tension and viscosity. Increasing the voltage beyond the threshold for jet initiation increases the degree of whipping instability and hence the elongation of the fibre jet. However, on the other hand, it also reduces the flight time between the spinneret and the collector. Hence, its effect on the fibre products is controversial. While numerous studies have observed decreasing fibre diameter with increasing applied voltage,[29] many others have shown minimal effect or an increase in fibre diameter.[30]

This discrepancy in the literature is a result of the interrelationship between applied voltage and other parameters such as flow rate and collection distance. If the voltage is too high and the flow rate is sufficient to maintain an increased rate of mass transfer, then multiple jets may be formed from the Taylor cone. This should be avoided, because it can lead to the products comprising several different subpopulations of polydisperse fibres. Voltage is therefore an important parameter, but no general statements can be made, other than to say it must be greater than V_k, the critical voltage needed to overcome the surface tension and emit a jet, and not so high as to lead to multiple jets forming or deplete the cone-shaped droplet at the nozzle exit.

In the majority of cases, a positive voltage is applied to the spinneret. Electrospinning with a negative voltage is also possible (as indeed is alternating current (AC) electrospinning, where the voltage alternates from positive to negative values), but both are much less explored than the positive polarity set-up. Studies have shown that AC current can cause non-uniform fibre diameters, and a negative polarity at the spinneret can result in fibres with larger average diameters.[15, 31]

Flow rate: Flow rate, also known as infusion rate or feed rate, is the rate at which the polymer solution is pumped into the spinneret to feed the spinning cone jet. The rate at which the solution is ejected from the spinneret collectively depends on the inner size of the spinneret orifice, the applied voltage (which provides the electrical force pulling the solution out of the needle) and the flow rate at which the solution is fed into the needle. As mentioned earlier, the voltage required for jet initiation is in turn dependent on the polymer solution properties. Therefore, at any given voltage, an optimum range of flow rates exists for a polymer material, which varies with the inner diameter of the needle. Fibre diameter increases and uniformity decreases with flow rates higher than this optimum range; a higher than optimum flow rate may not provide enough time for the polymer solution to become sufficiently charged to generate the Taylor cone, and some droplets may form upon exiting the spinneret.

A faster flow rate will usually lead to thicker fibres at a given voltage, because more mass is dispensed in a given unit of time. It may also produce fibres with defects such as beads or wrinkles if the solvent does not have time to evaporate completely before reaching the collector. Multiple jets can additionally be initiated if the flow rate is too high. On the other hand, at flow rates lower than the optimum range, electrospinning becomes discontinuous as the cone at the tip of the nozzle becomes depleted and even recedes into the needle.

Reducing the flow rate, of course, also has the disadvantage of increasing the time required to produce the desired amount of material. Hence, balancing the flow rate and applied voltage is vital in obtaining and maintaining a stable cone jet during electrospinning. To ensure steady mass transfer and continuous fibre production, the mass of liquid supplied to the needle tip needs to be equivalent to the mass of the jet spinning out of the needle.[32]

Spinneret: Metal spinnerets are most commonly used. In general, these comprise needles with small inner orifice diameters to generate narrow fibres.[33] The single-bore needles used for electrospinning monolithic fibres usually have diameters below 2 mm. A narrower-bore needle can be helpful in reducing the fibre diameter and also in preventing the formation of beaded fibres, but is also more prone to becoming blocked.

Spinneret-to-collector distance: The shorter this distance, the higher the electric field strength will be. However, the flight time will reduce with distance, and short distances can hence lead to incomplete solvent evaporation and the concomitant problems discussed in section 2.4.4. The optimum range for collection distance is most commonly 100–200 mm for conventional set-ups. Special apparatus such as near-field electrospinning, which requires a much lower collection distance, will be discussed in Chapter 6. Longer distances have been reported to lead to narrower fibres, because a greater period of elongation is possible. However, long distances beyond the optimum collection range will cause significant increases in the flight time, which can result in increased corona discharge and Rayleigh instability, leading to large fibre diameters and defects such as fused or beaded fibres.[34] For example, when increasing the collection distance from 10 to 30 cm, Kidoaki *et al.* (2006) observed a steady increase in fibre diameter from electrospun polyurethane in tetrahydrofuran and DMF mixed solvents.[34]

Finally, it is important to note that the polymer jet will discharge itself at the earliest opportunity, and thus using long distances can result in low yields and thinner fibre mats because the product is deposited over a larger surface of the collector, and in some cases not on the collector at all, but rather on the walls of the electrospinning chamber.

2.5.3 Environmental parameters

Environmental parameters are in essence the temperature and humidity of the location in which electrospinning takes place. It is also worth noting the surrounding speed of air flow: the presence of fast movements or changes in the degree of ventilation in the laboratory could affect the stability of the cone jet and the rate of solvent evaporation, leading to changes in the products obtained. To ensure reproducibility, it is usually best to conduct electrospinning in a space enclosed with an electrically insulating material such as plastic sheets.

An increase in humidity from 20% to 40% can reduce the as-spun fibre diameter, depending on the particular solvent used. This is because the evaporation rate of a solvent from a free surface is proportional to the difference between the vapour pressure of the solvent and the vapour pressure in the surrounding air. Increasing humidity retards the rate of solvent evaporation, thereby allowing longer time for fibre elongation. However, high humidities (> 60%)[35] can be problematic and often result in the formation of a film or poorly defined fused fibres on the collector, particularly with hygroscopic polymers such as poly(vinylpyrroli-done).[35a] This is because the absorption of water is favoured by a higher humidity and the concomitant greater partial pressure of water in the atmosphere; the presence of such high amounts of water in the air excessively retards the rate of solvent evaporation, allowing wet fibres to land on the collector and the possibility for this atmospheric water to interact with the products. If the polymer is insoluble in water it may precipitate in high-humidity environments, which can lead to blocking of the spinneret, thicker fibres, porosity or defects driven by phase separation in the products.

Higher temperatures will generate two opposing effects in electrospinning: on the one hand, it provides more energy to the molecules in solution, thereby increasing the electrical conductivity and reducing viscosity and surface tension of the solution. This facilitates the formation of finer fibre diameters as well as leading to higher polymer chain alignment (enhancing mechanical properties).[36] However, an increase in temperature also provides additional energy to accelerate the rate of solvent evaporation, reducing the time available for fibre elongation before solidification. Increasing the temperature from the ambient temperature of *ca.* 20°C to 40°C leads to reduced fibre diameter,[35a, 37] indicating that the former effect dominates over this temperature range. Fibre diameter was found to increase at temperatures higher than 40°C, however, indicating that here the faster solvent evaporation factor has overtaken the effect on surface tension and viscosity. There is very limited literature on the effect of temperatures cooler than the ambient temperature of approximately 20°C. However, Vrieze *et al.* observed reduced fibre diameters at 10°C and attributed this to a reduced rate of solvent evaporation.[35a]

2.5.4 Solvent and polymer selection

Pillay *et al.* have published an excellent review including the typical parameter ranges used for the electrospinning of a range of polymers for drug delivery purposes.[38] A summary is given in Tables 2.1 and 2.2.

2.6 The experimental set-up

The equipment needed for electrospinning will be briefly introduced in this section. More detail will be presented in subsequent chapters where the different types of electrospinning are discussed.

2.6.1 Basics

As discussed in section 2.3, the basic electrospinning apparatus consists of a high-voltage power supply, syringe pump, syringe fitted with a spinneret and a collector. All of these can be purchased at relatively low cost, and it is possible to construct a home-made set-up for a few thousand dollars (certainly less than $4000). Alternatively, a range of ready-made commercial apparatus exists, for instance from YFlow,[39] SprayBase,[40] or IME Technologies.[41] These are more expensive, ranging from around $15,000 to more than $100,000, but have advantages in terms of ease of getting the equipment up and running and access to specialist advice, of particular benefit to groups working on electrospinning for the first time.

There are two ways of setting up the orientation between the spinneret and the collector in electrospinning: vertically or horizontally.

Table 2.1 The properties of some solvents commonly used in the preparation of electrospun drug delivery systems

Solvent	*Boiling point (°C)*	*Other properties*	*Fibre morphology*	*References*
Dichloromethane	39.8	Low dielectric constant, high surface tension	Beaded, large diameter	*J. Biomater. Sci.* 2006, 17, 9, 1039 *J. Polym. Sci. B* 2004, 42, 20, 3721
Chloroform	61.2	High intrinsic viscosity	Beaded at very low polymer concentration, smooth at higher concentration	*Polymer* 2004, 45, 9, 2959
Methanol	64.7	High dielectric constant	Small fibre diameter with dichloromethane/methanol mixtures until the methanol concentration reached 50%, then rising fibre diameter	*J. Biomater. Sci.* 2006, 17, 9, 1039
Tetrahydrofuran	66	High dipole moment, good conductivity	Smooth and beaded, ribbon-like, high pore density	*Polymer* 220, 43, 16, 4403 *Eur. Polym. J.* 2005, 41, 3, 409
Ethyl acetate	77.1	High dielectric constant, fair conductivity	Smooth and beaded, ribbon-like	*Eur. Polym. J.* 2005, 41, 3, 409
Ethanol	78.3	Low surface tension, high intrinsic viscosity	Smooth, large diameter	*Polymer* 1999, 40, 16, 4585 *J. Polym. Sci. B* 2004, 42, 20, 3721 *Polymer* 2004, 45, 9, 2959
Methyl ethyl ketone	79.6	High dipole moment, good conductivity	Flat, ribbon-like, very few beads	*Eur. Polym. J.* 2005, 41, 3, 409

Dichloroethane	83.5	High dipole moment, fair conductivity	Smooth and beaded, C-shaped	*Eur. Polym. J.* 2005, 41, 3, 409
Water	100	Low intrinsic viscosity	Beaded, small diameter	*Polymer* 1999, 40, 16, 4585 *Polymer* 2004, 45, 9, 2959
Dimethyl formamide	153	High dipole moment, high conductivity, low intrinsic viscosity	Smooth and beaded, round	*Polymer* 2004, 45, 9, 2959 *Eur. Polym. J.* 2005, 41, 3, 409

Adapted with permission from Pillay, V.; Dott, C.; Choonara, Y. E.; Tyagi, C.; Tomar, L.; Kumar, P.; du Toit, L. C.; Ndesendo, V. M. K. 'A review of the effect of processing variables on the fabrication of electrospun nanofibers for drug delivery applications.' *J. Nanomater.* 2013 (2013): 789289.

Table 2.2 Polymers and solvent types commonly used in the preparation of electrospun drug delivery systems, together with examples of the drugs which have been incorporated

Polymer	*Solvent*	*Active ingredient(s)*	*References*
Cellulose acetate	2:1 acetone/ dimethylacetamide	Naproxen, indomethacin, ibuprofen, sulindac	*Polymer* 2007, 48, 17, 5030
		Curcumin	*Polymer* 2007, 48, 26, 7546
		Vitamins A and E	*Eur. J. Pharm. Biopharm.* 2007, 67, 2, 387
Poly(ε-caprolactone)	7:3 dichloromethane/ methanol	Heparin	*Biomater*. 2006, 27, 9, 2042
	3:1 chloroform/ethanol	Resveratrol, gentamicin	*J. Biomed. Mater. Res. A* 2006, 77, 1, 169
Poly(ethylene oxide)/poly(ε-caprolactone) blend	Chloroform	Lysozyme	*Colloids Surf. A* 2008, 313–314, 183
Poly(vinyl alcohol)	Deionised water	Ketoprofen	*Mater. Sci. Eng. A* 2007, 459, 1–2, 390
		Sodium salicylate, diclofenac, naproxen, indomethacin	*Nanotechnol*. 2006, 17, 9, 2317
Gelatin/poly(vinyl alcohol) blend	Gelatin in formic acid, poly(vinyl alcohol) in deionised water	Raspberry ketone	*Carbohydrate Polym.* 2007, 69, 3, 538
Poly(lactic-co-glycolic acid)	Dichloromethane/ dimethyl formamide	Paclitaxel	*Biomater*. 2008, 29, 20, 2996
	Dimethyl formamide	Cefoxitin sodium	*J. Control. Release* 2004, 98, 1, 47

Polyurethane	Dimethyl formamide	Itraconazole	*J. Control. Release* 2003, 92, 3, 349
	Dimethylacetamide	Ketanserin	
Poly(L-lactic acid)	2:1 chloroform/acetone	Doxorubicin HCl	*J. Control. Release* 2005, 105, 1–2, 43
		Tetracycline HCl	*J. Macromol. Sci. B* 2006, 45, 4, 515
	Chloroform	Cytochrome *c*	*J. Control. Release* 2008, 127, 2, 180
	Dichloromethane	Bovine serum albumin	*Biomacromol.* 2006, 7, 8, 2327
Poly(ethylene-co-vinylacetate)	Chloroform	Tetracycline HCl	*J. Control. Release* 2002, 81, 1–2, 57
Poly(ethylene glycol)–poly(L-lactic acid) copolymer	Chloroform	Doxorubicin HCl	*Eur. J. Pharm. Biopharm.* 2008, 70, 1, 165 *J. Control. Release* 2005, 108, 1, 33
Poly(acrylic acid)/poly(allylamine hydrochloride) blend	Deionised water	Methylene blue	*Colloids Surf. B* 2007, 58, 2, 172

Adapted with permission from Pillay, V.; Dott, C.; Choonara, Y. E.; Tyagi, C.; Tomar, L.; Kumar, P.; du Toit, L. C.; Ndesendo, V. M. K. 'A review of the effect of processing variables on the fabrication of electrospun nanofibers for drug delivery applications.' *J. Nanomater.* 2013 (2013): 789289.

The difference lies simply in the direction of liquid travel: in the former approach, liquid is dispensed in a direction perpendicular to the floor and aided by gravity, while in the latter it travels parallel to it. Both have advantages and disadvantages. In the horizontal approach, the force of gravity on the fluid jet can become significant if the collection distance is greater than 10 cm, and the jet can be dragged downwards, away from the collecting area, as a result. This can cause fibres to build up at the bottom of the collector, or even below it, compromising the effective yield of the process. In the vertical approach, gravity is acting in the same direction as the electrostatic accelerating force. However, the downside of the vertical approach is that, if any droplets are formed during the process (e.g. when pausing or restarting the process), these can potentially fall on to the collector, compromising the quality of the products. In the horizontal approach, the droplets will fall to the bottom of the experimental chamber and will not reach the collector, and thus the product can be of higher quality.

2.6.2 The power supply and syringe pump

These are commercial items which can be purchased from a large number of different suppliers. The major issues to consider when buying are the cost vs. the precision and stability of the power supply and pumps, and whether the apparatus meets the user's needs in terms of the range of voltages which the supply will generate and the rates at which the pump will dispense. In general, a simple power supply capable of producing a positive voltage up to 25 kV should suffice (most electrospinning is performed between around 5 and 25 kV).

2.6.3 The spinneret

In the simplest electrospinning experiment, termed *monoaxial* electrospinning, a solution of a polymer and drug is dispensed through a single-bore blunt-end needle, most often made of a conductive and solvent-resistant metal such as stainless steel. This gives a monolithic product, with the drug and polymer typically evenly and homogeneously blended throughout the fibres. However, it is possible to process two, three or even more liquids as compound jets (co-flowing liquid jets) and a range of more complicated spinnerets such as concentric or multi-needle designs can be prepared to generate sophisticated nanostructures made of multiple polymers and/or active pharmaceutical ingredients. A summary of the most important designs is given in Figure 2.8. To process multiple liquids, each is loaded into a separate syringe and dispensed independently using multiple syringe pumps.

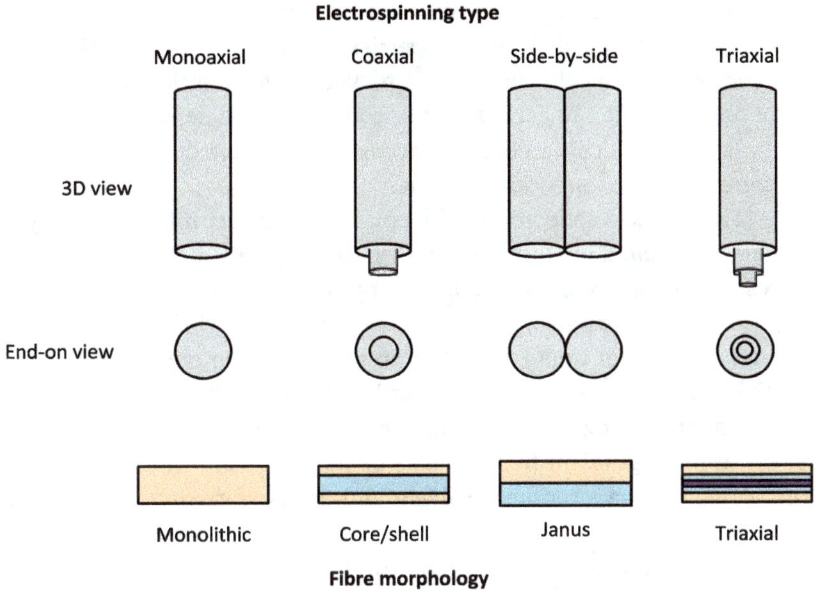

Figure 2.8 Spinneret designs for different types of electrospinning, and the structures of the fibres produced.

Coaxial electrospinning uses a coaxial needle that contains two capillary channels arranged in a concentric manner. Each channel is infused with a polymer solution at an individual flow rate. If the experiment is well designed and optimised there will be minimal blending between the two solutions, and since the electrospinning process is very fast the concentric structure of the spinneret will result in core/shell fibres with two distinct compartments (Figure 2.8). Similarly, if two needles are arranged *side by side* the fibres produced should have a Janus morphology, with two different sides. Moving up to three or four liquids can yield three-layer or even four-layer fibres if a triaxial or quad-axial concentric spinneret is used. There are a range of more complicated spinneret designs but the key types of electrospinning as far as this volume is concerned are monoaxial, coaxial, triaxial/quad-axial, and side-by-side; they will be discussed in more detail in subsequent chapters.

2.6.4 The collector

The speed at which each layer of the produced nanofibres becomes discharged upon reaching the collector plays a significant role in controlling the spacing and density of the fibre mat. This discharging process is affected by the dielectric properties, surface area and the collective conductivity of the collecting substrate. Various geometries of collectors have been designed to achieve better control of fibre deposition density and alignment. A comprehensive review on collector designs has been undertaken by Teo and Ramakrishna.[42]

The simplest collector is a flat conducting collector plate, usually a metal plate coated in aluminium foil. This will give a mat of non-woven fibres which are randomly oriented. For most drug delivery applications, this is perfectly satisfactory. However, a problem can arise when spinning for long periods of time (> 2 h) to prepare larger amounts of product. As the layer of fibres on the collector builds up and becomes thicker, it acts as an insulating coating to the grounded collector. This reduces the electrical field gradient to new fibres being deposited, which can result in incomplete evaporation of solvent and defects forming at the top of the mat.

It can thus sometimes be useful to employ a rotating mandrel collector. This increases the area of fibres which can be collected, and is depicted in Figure 2.9. Here, the collector comprises a conducting cylinder which rotates along its long axis. To ensure even coverage of the collector, the spinneret is moved back and forth along the length (*rastering*). This generates a tubular structure. At the end of the experiment, a scalpel can be used to cut through and remove the fibres as a flat mat. If the tube can be rolled off the mandrel without damaging it, the rotating mandrel set-up can be used to prepare tubular scaffolds for tissue engineering, for instance of veins or arteries.[43]

With the recent explosion of interest in electrospinning technology, a number of more sophisticated collecting systems have been reported.

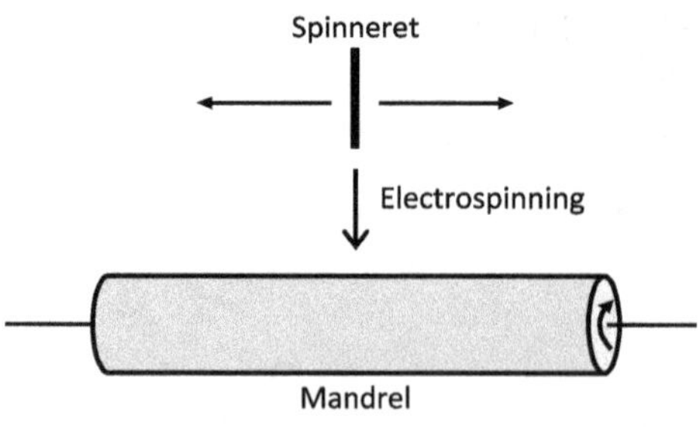

Figure 2.9 A schematic showing the use of a rotating mandrel collector with a rastering spinneret.

For instance, for tissue-engineering scaffolds it can often be desirable to obtain aligned fibres. This can be achieved by rotating a cylindrical mandrel very quickly (at a rate of hundreds or thousands of revolutions per second). Alternatively, a collector comprising parallel electrodes can be used to achieve alignment. For the purposes of drug delivery systems, alignment is not generally necessary, however, and the majority of the examples discussed in this volume use simple flat-plate detectors. When scaling electrospinning up for industrial applications, conveyor belt-type collectors are required to allow continuous manufacturing; we will discuss these more in Chapter 7.

2.6.5 Other considerations

Most commonly, research on electrospinning is carried out in laboratories on the benchtop. Care must be taken when doing this because many of the solvents used for preparing polymer solutions smell unpleasant, and some are harmful. A robust risk assessment is thus required, but because the volumes of solvents used are small and the dispensing rates low there are normally no problems spinning in a well-ventilated laboratory. However, because humidity, temperature and the surrounding speed of air flow have a major influence on the electrospinning process, the ambient conditions and the location of experiment need to be monitored and recorded throughout to ensure it can be reproduced. Equipment exists which can precisely control temperature and humidity, but this often costs more than $5000 and requires a large isolated space (around 2 m^3) to house the cumbersome and bulky apparatus. Both these factors are usually highly inconvenient for many research labs. A simpler alternative is to procure a simple temperature and humidity meter and monitor these quantities throughout experiments to ensure reproducibility.

When preparing polymer solutions for spinning it is necessary to ensure that the polymer fully dissolves in the solvent to yield a solution with appropriate properties (in terms of conductivity and viscosity). Achieving this can require extensive optimisation. Solution preparation, together with other important considerations for a successful experiment, will be considered in detail in Chapters 3–5 as they differ somewhat for the different spinning processes.

2.6.6 Establishing and troubleshooting an electrospinning process

A more detailed discussion of how to set up and optimise fibre production will be provided in Chapters 3–5 for single-fluid, coaxial and triaxial, and side-by-side processes, respectively. An excellent overview of the steps to be followed can be found in an instructive video article by Leach *et al.*[44]

2.7 Fibre properties

The fibres produced by electrospinning can be made from a wide variety of polymers, with very different drug release properties. For instance, the use of a fast-dissolving polymer such as PEO can accelerate the rate at which a drug gets into solution. Alternatively, a slow-dissolving or water-insoluble polymer such as poly(lactic-co-glycolic acid) or poly(ε-caprolactone) will give extended release, while a pH-sensitive polymer such as poly(methacrylic acid-co-methyl methacrylate) can be employed to target release to the small intestine by exploiting the changes in pH in the different parts of the body. Complicated architectures can be prepared through multi-liquid processing, and the diameter, porosity and mechanical properties of the fibre mat can all be tuned by systematic variation of material and processing parameters. These properties all lead to the products of electrospinning having a wide range of potential applications in the drug delivery field.

2.8 Characterisation

As described in detail in section 1.4, the first characterisation performed on an electrospun product is generally a simple visual inspection of a few fibres collected on a glass slide. If fibres can clearly be seen, then they can be inspected under a microscope to check if the process is optimised (are the fibres linear, or are beads present? Are there any particles or droplets present?). Once small quantities of good-quality fibres have been prepared, a larger batch can be produced. Typical characterisation for this would include scanning electron microscopy to check the fibre morphology, with transmission electron microscopy, focused ion beam microscopy and/or confocal microscopy often also undertaken to check for internal structure, particularly in the case of fibres from coaxial or multi-axial spinning. The ImageJ software (freely available from https://imagej.nih.gov/ij/) can be employed to quantify the fibre diamaters. The physical form of the drug and polymer is usually investigated with X-ray diffraction and differential scanning calorimetry, and infrared spectroscopy is used to study the functional groups present in the fibres and any interactions between components. Thermogravimetric analysis can be performed to check for the presence of any residual solvent in the fibres; if solvent does remain and this is problematic, then the fibres can be stored in a desiccator or vacuum oven to remove this.

Depending on the intended application, it may be necessary to evaluate the mechanical properties of the fibres, and in the majority of cases drug release will be quantified through dissolution experiments. Permeation studies and *in vivo* work may also be appropriate if all the previous assays give promising results.

2.9 Summary

In this chapter, the EHD process has been introduced and explained. A brief discussion of the fundamental physics behind electrospinning has been presented, followed by a detailed discussion of the parameters which can affect the process and the nature of the influence they have. The requirements to establish a successful electrospinning experiment to generate defect-free fibres have been described. As a result, the reader should now have a good grasp of the overarching principles of electrospinning. Subsequent chapters will describe the different processes in more detail and explore the applications of the fibres produced.

2.10 References

1. (a) Reneker, D. H.; Yarin, A. L. 'Electrospinning jets and polymer nanofibers.' *Polymer* 49 (2008): 2387–2425; (b) Luo, C. J.; Stoyanov, S. D.; Stride, E.; Pelan, E.; Edirisinghe, M. 'Electrospinning versus fibre production methods: from specifics to technological convergence.' *Chem. Soc. Rev.* 41 (2012): 4708–4735.
2. Cooley, J. F. Improved methods of and apparatus for electrically separating the relatively volatile liquid component from the component of relatively fixed substances of composite fluids. Patent number GB 06385, 1900.
3. (a) Zeleny, J. 'Instability of electrified liquid surfaces.' *Phys. Rev.* 10 (1917): 1–6; (b) Zeleny, J. 'The electrical discharge from liquid points, and a hydrostatic method of measuring the electric intensity at their surfaces.' *Phys. Rev.* 7 (1914): 69–91.
4. Formhals, A. Process and apparatus for preparing artificial threads. Patent number US 1975504, 1934.

5. Formhals, A. Method and apparatus for spinning. Patent number US 2160962, 1939.
6. Filatov, Y.; Budyka, A.; Kirichenko, V., *Electrospinning of Micro- and Nanofibers: Fundamentals and applications in separation and filtration processes.* New York: Begell House, 2007.
7. (a) Taylor, G. 'Disintegration of water drops in an electric field.' *Proc. R. Soc. Lond. A* 280 (1964): 383–397; (b) Taylor, G. I. 'Electrically driven jets.' *Proc. R. Soc. A* 313 (1969): 453–475.
8. Simons, H. L. Process and apparatus for producing patterned non-woven fabrics. Patent number US 3280229, 1966.
9. (a) Larrondo, L.; Manley, R. S. J. 'Electrostatic fiber spinning from polymer melts. I. Experimental observations on fiber formation and properties.' *J. Polym. Sci. B: Polym. Phys.* 19 (1981): 909–920; (b) Cooley, J. F. Apparatus for electrically dispersing fluids. Patent number US 692631, 1902.
10. Doshi, J.; Reneker, D. H. Electrospinning process and applications of electrospun fibers. In *Proceedings IEEE-Ind. Appl. Soc. Annual Meeting*, Toronto, Canada, 1993; pp. 1698–1703.
11. (a) Fong, H.; Chun, I.; Reneker, D. H. 'Beaded nanofibers formed during electrospinning.' *Polymer* 40 (1999): 4585–4592; (b) Reneker, D. H.; Chun, I. 'Nanometre diameter fibres of polymer, produced by electrospinning.' *Nanotechnology* 7 (1996): 216–223; (c) Reneker, D. H.; Yarin, A. L.; Fong, H.; Koombhongse, S. 'Bending instability of electrically charged liquid jets of polymer solutions in electrospinning.' *J. Appl. Phys.* 87 (2000): 4531–4747.
12. Xie, J.; Jiang, J.; Davoodi, P.; Srinivasan, M. P.; Wang, C. H. 'Electrohydrodynamic atomization: A two-decade effort to produce and process micro-/nanoparticulate materials.' *Chem. Eng. Sci.* 125 (2015): 32–57.
13. He, X.-X.; Zheng, J.; Yu, G.-F.; You, M.-H.; Yu, M.; Ning, X.; Long, Y.-Z. 'Near-field electrospinning: Progress and applications.' *J. Phys. Chem. C* 121 (2017): 8663–8678.
14. (a) Sill, T. J.; von Recum, H. A. 'Electrospinning: Applications in drug delivery and tissue engineering.' *Biomaterials* 29 (2008): 1989–2006; (b) Villarreal-Gómez, L. J.; Cornejo-Bravo, J. M.; Vera-Graziano, R.; Grande, D. 'Electrospinning as a powerful technique for biomedical applications: a critically selected survey.' *J. Biomater. Sci. Polym. Ed.* 27 (2016): 157–176.
15. Mit-uppatham, C.; Nithitanakul, M.; Supaphol, P. 'Effects of solution concentration, emitting electrode polarity, solvent type, and salt addition on electrospun polyamide-6 fibers: A preliminary report.' *Macromol. Symp.* 216 (2004): 293–299.
16. Garg, K.; Bowlin, G. L. 'Electrospinning jets and nanofibrous structures.' *Biomicrofluidics* 5 (2011): 013403.
17. Rangkupan, R.; Reneker, D. H. 'Electrospinning process of molten polypropylene in vacuum.' *J. Met. Mater. Miner.* 12 (2003): 81–87.

18. MacDiarmid, A. G.; Jones Jr, W. E.; Norris, I. D.; Gao, J.; Johnson Jr, A. T.; Pinto, N. J.; Hone, J.; Han, B.; Ko, F. K.; Okuzaki, H.; Llaguno, M. 'Electrostatically-generated nanofibers of electronic polymers.' *Synth. Met.* 119 (2001): 37–40.
19. Watanabe, H. 'Viscoelasticity and dynamics of entangled polymers.' *Prog. Polym. Sci.* 24 (1999): 1253–1403.
20. Cloupeau, M.; Prunetfoch, B. 'Electrostatic spraying of liquids – main functioning modes.' *J. Electrost.* 25 (1990): 165–184.
21. Doshi, J.; Reneker, D. H. 'Electrospinning process and applications of electrospun fibers.' *J. Electrost.* 35 (1995): 151–160.
22. Shenoy, S. L.; Bates, W. D.; Frisch, H. L.; Wnek, G. E. 'Role of chain entanglements on fiber formation during electrospinning of polymer solutions: Good solvent, non-specific polymer–polymer interaction limit.' *Polymer* 46 (2005): 3372–3384.
23. Yang, Q.; Li, Z.; Hong, Y.; Zhao, Y.; Qiu, S.; Wang, C.; Wei, Y. 'Influence of solvents on the formation of ultrathin uniform poly(vinyl pyrrolidone) nanofibers with electrospinning.' *J. Polym. Sci. B: Polym. Phys.* 42 (2004): 3721–3726.
24. Koski, A.; Yim, K.; Shivkumar, S. 'Effect of molecular weight on fibrous PVA produced by electrospinning.' *Mater. Lett.* 58 (2004): 493–497.
25. Baumgarten, P. K. 'Electrostatic spinning of acrylic microfibers.' *J. Colloid Interface Sci.* 36 (1971): 71–79.
26. Morota, K.; Matsumoto, H.; Mizukoshi, T.; Konosu, Y.; Minagawa, M.; Tanioka, A.; Yamagata, Y.; Inoue, K. 'Poly(ethylene oxide) thin films produced by electrospray deposition: Morphology control and additive effects of alcohols on nanostructure.' *J. Colloid Interface Sci.* 279 (2004): 484–492.
27. (a) Wannatong, L.; Sirivat, A.; Supaphol, P. 'Effects of solvents on electrospun polymeric fibers: Preliminary study on polystyrene.' *Polym. Int.* 53 (2004): 1851–1859; (b) Son, W. K.; Youk, J. H.; Lee, T. S.; Park, W. H. 'The effects of solution properties and polyelectrolyte on electrospinning of ultrafine poly(ethylene oxide) fibers.' *Polymer* 45 (2004): 2959–2966; (c) Luo, C. J.; Stride, E.; Edirisinghe, M. 'Mapping the influence of solubility and dielectric constant on electrospinning polycaprolactone solutions.' *Macromolecules* 45 (2012): 4669–4680.
28. Luo, C. J.; Nangrejo, M.; Edirisinghe, M. 'A novel method of selecting solvents for polymer electrospinning.' *Polymer* 51 (2010): 1654–1662.
29. (a) Fridrikh, S. V.; Yu, J. H.; Brenner, M. P.; Rutledge, G. C. 'Controlling the fiber diameter during electrospinning.' *Phys. Rev. Lett.* 90 (2003): 144502-1-4; (b) Megelski, S.; Stephens, J. S.; Chase, D. B.; Rabolt, J. F. 'Micro- and nanostructured surface morphology on electrospun polymer fibers.' *Macromol.* 35 (2002): 456–466.
30. (a) Gu, S. Y.; Ren, J.; Vancso, G. J. 'Process optimization and empirical modeling for electrospun polyacrylonitrile (PAN) nanofiber precursor of

carbon nanofibers.' *Eur. Polym. J.* 41 (2005): 2559–2568; (b) Tan, S.-H.; Inai, R.; Kotaki, M.; Ramakrishna, S. 'Systematic parameter study for ultra-fine fiber fabrication via electrospinning process.' *Polymer* 46 (2005): 6128–6134.

31. (a) Kalayci, V. E.; Patra, P. K.; Kim, Y. K.; Ugbolue, S. C.; Warner, S. B. 'Charge consequences in electrospun polyacrylonitrile (PAN) nanofibers.' *Polymer* 46 (2005): 7191–7200; (b) Supaphol, P.; Mit-Uppatham, C.; Nithitanakul, M. 'Ultrafine electrospun polyamide-6 fibers: Effect of emitting electrode polarity on morphology and average fiber diameter.' *J. Polym. Sci. B: Polym. Phys.* 43 (2005): 3699–3712.
32. Deitzel, J. M.; Kleinmeyer, J.; Harris, D.; Beck Tan, N. C. 'The effect of processing variables on the morphology of electrospun nanofibers and textiles.' *Polymer* 42 (2001): 261–272.
33. Katti, D. S.; Robinson, K. W.; Ko, F. K.; Laurencin, C. T. 'Bioresorbable nanofiber-based systems for wound healing and drug delivery: Optimization of fabrication parameters.' *J. Biomed. Mater. Res. B* 70B (2004): 286–296.
34. Kidoaki, S.; Kwon, K.; Matsuda, T. 'Structural features and mechanical properties of in situ-bonded meshes of segmented polyurethane electrospun from mixed solvents.' *J. Biomed. Mater. Res. B* 76B (2006): 219–229.
35. (a) Vrieze, S. D.; Camp, T. V.; Nelvig, A.; Hagström, B.; Westbroek, P.; Clerck, K. D. 'The effect of temperature and humidity on electrospinning.' *J. Mater. Sci.* 44 (2009): 1357; (b) Pelipenko, J.; Kristl, J.; Janković, B.; Baumgartner, S.; Kocbek, P. 'The impact of relative humidity during electrospinning on the morphology and mechanical properties of nanofibers.' *Int. J. Pharm.* 456 (2013): 125–134.
36. Wang, C.; Chien, H.-S.; Hsu, C.-H.; Wang, Y.-C.; Wang, C.-T.; Lu, H.-A. 'Electrospinning of polyacrylonitrile solutions at elevated temperatures.' *Macromol.* 40 (2007): 7973–7983.
37. Yang, G. Z.; Li, H. P.; Yang, J. H.; Wan, J.; Yu, D. G. 'Influence of working temperature on the formation of electrospun polymer nanofibers.' *Nanoscale Res. Lett.* 12 (2017): 55.
38. Pillay, V.; Dott, C.; Choonara, Y. E.; Tyagi, C.; Tomar, L.; Kumar, P.; du Toit, L. C.; Ndesendo, V. M. K. 'A review of the effect of processing variables on the fabrication of electrospun nanofibers for drug delivery applications.' *J. Nanomater.* 2013 (2013): 789289.
39. www.yflow.com/. Accessed 25 June 2017.
40. www.spraybase.com/. Accessed 25 June 2017.
41. www.imetechnologies.com/. Accessed 25 June 2017.
42. Teo, W. E.; Ramakrishna, S. 'A review on electrospinning design and nanofibre assemblies.' *Nanotechnology* 17 (2006): R89–R106.
43. (a) Nottelet, B.; Pektok, E.; Mandracchia, D.; Tille, J. C.; Walpoth, B.; Gurny, R.; Moller, M. 'Factorial design optimization and *in vivo* feasibility of poly(epsilon-caprolactone)-micro- and nanofiber-based small diameter

vascular grafts.' *J. Biomed. Mater. Res. A* 89 (2009): 865–875; (b) Hajiali, H.; Shahgasempour, S.; Naimi-Jamal, M. R.; Peirovi, H. 'Electrospun PGA/gelatin nanofibrous scaffolds and their potential application in vascular tissue engineering.' *Int. J. Nanomedicine* 6 (2011): 2133–2141.

44. Leach, M. K.; Z.Q., F.; Tuck, S. J.; Corey, J. M. 'Electrospinning fundamentals: Optimizing solution and apparatus parameters.' *J. Vis. Exp.* 47 (2011): e2494.

3

A Complete Study of Monoaxial Electrospinning

3.1 Introduction

Monoaxial (or uniaxial) electrospinning is the simplest route by which fibres can be made using the electrohydrodynamic technique. To employ this to generate drug delivery systems, a mixed liquid (solution, emulsion or suspension) of a polymer and a drug in a (typically volatile) solvent is first prepared. This is dispensed through a single-bore blunt-end needle (often made of a solvent-resistant metal such as stainless steel) towards a metal collector (such as a stainless steel plate or an aluminium sheet), with a high electrical potential difference (commonly 5–20 kV for monoaxial single-liquid electrospinning) applied between the two. The fibres collected comprise monolithic systems, with the drug most usually evenly dispersed throughout the polymer, as depicted in Figure 3.1. Because the electrospinning process is very rapid, with the time between the solution exiting the spinneret and reaching the collector being well under a second, the arrangement of the molecules in the solution is propagated into the solid state. Thus, electrospun fibres typically take the form of amorphous solid dispersions (ASDs), as described in section 1.3.4.

The first report of electrospun fibres being used in the drug delivery context came from Kenawy *et al.*[1] These researchers generated fibres loaded with tetracycline hydrochloride using poly(lactic acid) (PLA), poly(ethylene-co-vinyl acetate) (PEVA) or a blend of the two as the filament-forming polymer matrix. Since then, a vast number of studies have been reported in which fibres from electrospinning are explored for drug delivery: a Web of Science search for 'electrospinning

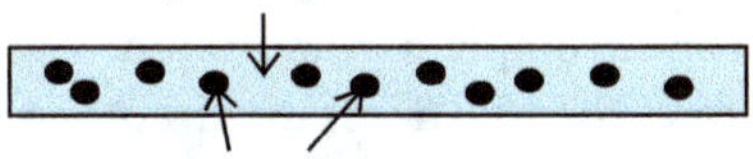

Figure 3.1 A schematic illustration of an electrospun fibre from monoaxial spinning.

AND drug delivery' on 28 June 2017 gave 1547 hits. This interest has arisen because there are a number of advantages of using electrospun nanofibres in drug delivery. These include: (1) high drug loadings (up to 60%) and encapsulation efficiency (up to 100%);[2] (2) a wide range of polymers (> 100) can be spun;[3] (3) drug release can be modulated through the choice of polymer (hydrophilic or hydrophobic, molecular weight);[4] (4) the fibres have high specific surface areas (10–100 $m^2\ g^{-1}$);[5] and (5) the process is simple to perform and cost-effective, on the laboratory scale at least.[6]

In this chapter, we will review the major applications of fibres from monoaxial spinning in drug delivery.

3.2 Experimental considerations

As was discussed in section 2.5, a number of solution and processing parameters need to be controlled for successful electrospinning.

3.2.1 Solution parameters

The molecular weight and concentration of the polymer(s) and the choice of solvent are important because they control the viscosity, surface tension and conductivity of the spinning solution, and thus how it behaves in electrospinning. The spinnable viscosity range varies with the polymer and solvent, but should be at least around 120 cP. In very-low-viscosity solutions, there will be insufficient polymer chain entanglements to produce fibres.[7] In contrast, if the viscosity is too high then the surface tension cannot easily be overcome. In both cases, the result can be droplets or particles forming rather than fibres.

The solvent used must be capable of dissolving the polymer of interest at an appropriate concentration to form fibres, and must possess a suitable volatility. A low-volatility solvent like water (boiling point (b.p.) 100°C) may fail to evaporate completely over the distance between the spinneret and the collector. When the fibres form, they will hence contain residual water owing to this incomplete evaporation. The residue solvent will subsequently evaporate from the fibres upon storage, resulting in ribbon-like (flattened) fibres, wrinkles on the fibre surface or fused fibres. On the other hand, a high-volatility solvent may evaporate very quickly, leading to larger fibre diameters (less time for elongation before solidification) and clogging of the spinneret (due to drying of the liquid at the spinneret before jetting, or drying of the Taylor cone during jetting). Solvents commonly used for electrospinning include ethanol (b.p. 78°C), chloroform (61°C), dichloromethane (40°C) and hexafluoroisopropanol (58°C).

Mixtures of miscible solvents can be used to ensure that sufficient polymer can be dissolved to give a solution of appropriate viscosity and volatility with a suitable dielectric constant range to allow fibre formation. For instance, less volatile solvents such as dimethyl formamide (DMF: b.p. 153°C) and dimethylacetamide (b.p. 165°C) are frequently used in combination with more volatile solvents like acetone (b.p. 56°C), dichloromethane (b.p. 40°C), tetrahydrofuran (b.p. 66°C) or methanol (b.p. 64°C). However, care must be taken because using a mixture of solvents with very different volatilities can result in porous fibre structures, as reported by Katsogiannis *et al.* for organic solvent mixtures with dimethyl sulfoxide (DMSO).[8] DMSO evaporates much more slowly than the organic solvents used, which results in its incorporation into the fibres. The remaining DMSO will eventually evaporate, yielding porous fibres.

It is also important to take into account the surface tension of the solution. Solvents with very high surface tensions (e.g. water) can result in instability arising during the spinning process, and a broad range of fibre diameters in the products and/or the generation of electrosprayed particles rather than fibres. If necessary, a surfactant can be added to reduce the surface tension, but this will be incorporated into the fibres produced and may require post-spinning removal.

3.2.2 Processing parameters

The applied voltage needs to be sufficient to overcome the surface tension of the liquids being processed, giving a clear Taylor cone and emitting a polymer jet from the latter. The range of voltages suitable for monoaxial electrospinning in a conventional benchtop apparatus is typically between 5 and 25 kV.

The distance between the needle and collector, the temperature, the humidity and the surrounding air flow can exert a major influence on the process, as discussed in section 2.5.3. It will be important to monitor both temperature and humidity during the experimental process to ensure reproducibility.

The distance between the spinneret and collector is usually in the range of 10–20 cm. It is possible to place the collector further away, but problems arise because the charged polymer jet seeks the nearest grounded surface on which to discharge. Thus, higher distances can lead to much of the fibre product landing in places other than the collector. If the distance is too short, there will be insufficient time for solvent evaporation and the fibres may fuse or become wrinkled when the residual solvent in the fibre subsequently diffuses out on the collector.

Finally, we should note that these parameters are not mutually exclusive, and that varying one will inevitably have an effect on others (for instance, an increased temperature will result in reduced surface tension and viscosity of the solution). This means that, although the electrospinning process is conceptually simple, its implementation requires some optimisation. A good understanding of the fundamentals of electrospinning (as described in Chapter 2) can significantly facilitate the optimisation process.

3.2.3 The spinneret

The spinneret for monoaxial spinning most commonly comprises a simple narrow-bore, blunt-end metal needle. The diameter of this needle can vary, but most commonly researchers work with internal diameters below 1 mm, with around 0.4–0.8 mm probably being most usual. This translates to needles of gauge 18–22. In general, this simple spinneret design can be used to achieve successful spinning. A blunt end rather than a tapered end for the needle exit is important as the size and size distribution of the products increase with an increase in needle tip angle. Blunt-ended needles can be procured commercially, or a disposable medical hypodermic needle can be adapted by cutting off the bevelled edge of the needle with a pair of scissors and using a filing paper to smooth the end. However, it should be noted that there will be some interactions between the solvent and polymer molecules in the solution and the metal surface of the spinneret. There will exist some attractive forces between these (e.g. between polar groups in the polymer and the electropositive metal surface), which can act counter to the drawing force of the electric field and can pull the polymer solution back into the spinneret. It has been found that coating the spinneret exterior in a non-conducting and non-stick polymer such as

Teflon can reduce these interactions.[9] As a result, the electrical energy can be more efficiently used to elongate and narrow the polymer jet, and narrower fibres can be produced. In addition, strong attractive forces between the polymer jet and a metal spinneret can result in fibres or other solid material becoming attached to the needle, leading to lower yields and potentially to blocking of the exit orifice. This effect too can be ameliorated using a Teflon coating. An epoxy coating can also be used to similar ends.[10]

3.2.4 Polymer choice

The choice of polymer will be largely dependent on the intended application. For instance, if a fast-dissolving drug delivery system is required, then a rapidly dissolving hydrophilic polymer such as poly(vinyl pyrrolidone) (PVP) or poly(ethylene oxide) (PEO) should be selected. For extended release, a slow-dissolving polymer (e.g. poly(ε-caprolactone) (PCL) or poly(lactic-co-glycolic acid) (PLGA)) or a water-insoluble system (e.g. ethyl cellulose (EC)) can be employed. This will be discussed in more detail in subsequent sections of this chapter.

Consideration must also be given to compatibility between the polymer and the drug of interest. For instance, if a hydrophilic polymer is being used to form fibres but the drug is very hydrophobic, phase separation is likely to occur, to minimise any hydrophobic/hydrophilic contacts. The fibres will thus be unstable, and their functional performance will change upon storage. Selecting a polymer which can form intermolecular interactions (such as hydrogen bonding, van der Waals forces) with the drug can help to prevent this. The literature refers often to *component compatibility*, by which it means the possibility of forming such interactions to prevent phase segregation and encourage long-term stability. Infrared spectroscopy can be helpful to identify intermolecular interactions, which are indicated by small shifts in peak positions (see section 1.4.4).

A solution of the polymer at an appropriate concentration will need to be prepared for spinning. The concentration range required will vary widely depending on the polymer and solvent (see description of the critical concentration c_e in section 2.5). By way of example, PEOs with Mw $\leq$ 300 kDa in chloroform or ethanol solvent can be spun from solutions of 3–4% w/v, while very-high-molecular-weight PVP solutions in ethanol (Mw = 1300 kDa) are typically 6–10% w/v,[11] and for the naturally occurring polymer shellac, very high concentrations of around 80% w/v are needed.

3.2.5 Starting experimental work

When beginning a new electrospinning experiment, the literature will be an invaluable source of guidance as to suitable experimental parameters to use. Working from these precedents, the best place to start is to prepare a range of polymer solutions in the solvent of interest (i.e. one that dissolves both the polymer and drug at appropriate concentrations). If the best solvent to use is not known, then a solvent screen to explore the solubility of the polymer in a range of solvents commonly used for electrospinning (e.g. acetone, ethanol, dichloromethane, DMF, chloroform, methanol) can be helpful. In the authors' personal experience, we have found that very many materials dissolve in the solvent hexafluoroisopropanol. However, this solvent is both expensive and toxic; if it is to be used then care must be taken to ensure there is no residual solvent in the fibres produced.

If a single solvent does not prove satisfactory – for instance, because the volatility or dielectric constant is inappropriate – then solvent mixtures may offer the opportunity to modulate the solution properties. If a solution can be prepared which is a viscous liquid but flows (that is, it is slightly sticky, like honey), then it is suitable for further study. If the polymer concentration is too high, then a gel will be obtained – this will not flow under gravity, and will not be spinnable.

Once a series of solutions has been prepared, electrospinning can begin. The solution should be loaded into a syringe, taking care to avoid any air bubbles. The spinneret is then fitted to the syringe, which is mounted on to the syringe pump. For viscous solutions, the experimenter may find it preferable to use a syringe with a Luer lock tip, which connects with the needle in a more secure fashion than slip tip syringes.

The solution should be dispensed slowly from the needle; 0.5–6 mL h^{-1} is a generally appropriate range. As an approximate guide to flow rate, when a droplet forms at the tip, wipe it away; if the droplet is immediately replaced then the flow rate is in an appropriate range for spinning.

The high-voltage power supply should now be connected to the needle with the mains power remaining switched off for safety, and the collector grounded. Next, increase the voltage slowly from zero until the Taylor cone can be seen, and a long jet of polymer is ejected from it. The process should now be monitored for a few minutes to see if the cone jet remains stable and continuous. If so, then optimisation of the processing parameters can begin in order to fine-tune the morphology and diameter of the fibres. If not, then the polymer concentration will need to be adjusted. This procedure is depicted in a video article by Leach and co-workers.[12]

It is important to take care when increasing the voltage beyond 18 kV. If the voltage is too high then the flow rate feeding the solution into the needle may not keep up with the electric field drawing the solution out of the needle, and the Taylor cone may disappear into the spinneret (see section 2.5.2 for a detailed description of the effect of processing parameters on the electrospun product).[13]

The next stage is to look at the fibres formed. To do this, we recommend collecting for around 5 s to 1 min on a glass slide or aluminium sheet, and then examining this under a microscope (see section 1.4.1 on nanofibre characterisation by microscopy). By systematically varying the voltage, flow rate and spinneret-to-collector distance from the initially identified parameters it should be possible to produce high-quality monodisperse fibres with a uniform morphology and diameter distribution and no beading or other defects (see sections 2.4 and 2.5).

3.3 Fibre properties

By varying the material and processing parameters, it is possible to obtain control of the surface morphology and porosity of the fibres generated. Their surface is generally smooth if the materials and processing parameters are optimised. A high electrical potential or low concentration tends to result in beaded structures with considerably rougher surfaces, however.[14] In very concentrated solutions, as well as the main population of fibres, a secondary population of smaller fibres is often seen.[15] The fibre diameter can be controlled by tuning the solution and processing parameters (e.g. polymer concentration, flow rate, voltage), as described in section 2.5.

Two types of pores are possible with the fibre mats generated by electrospinning. Pores may form on or within the fibres themselves, and there will also be pores between the layers of fibres forming the mat (unless the fibres are electrospun with a very high degree of alignment such as by direct writing melt electrospinning; see Chapter 6 for more details).[15b, 16] A knowledge of pore size and porosity can be important, because in many cases it will affect the performance of the formulation. The pore size will control the size of substances which can pass through the fibre mat (individual molecules will always be able to pass through, but cells require pores of tens of microns to permeate into the mat). The porosity will affect the diffusion rate across the fibre mat, governing for instance how rapidly water can penetrate into the aggregate of fibres and interact with the polymer and drug molecules.[15b] All these properties will influence the drug release profiles observed. If it is necessary to increase the porosity of the fibre mat, porogens (e.g. salt and clay particles) can be added to the polymer solution, and then removed after electrospinning. This usually leads to micron-sized pores where the porogens were originally situated.[17]

3.4 Some typical results

After electrospinning, the standard series of characterisations to be performed will comprise an assessment of the fibres using electron microscopy (to visualise morphology), together with X-ray diffraction (XRD) and differential scanning calorimetry (DSC) to observe physical form. Infrared spectroscopy will be employed to look for any interactions between the components of the fibres, and then functional performance studies will be undertaken (see sections 1.4 and 2.8). A typical set of results from one of our studies is given in Figure 3.2. These data are for PVP fibres loaded with indomethacin.[18] Materials were prepared with drug contents between 9.1% and 33.3% w/w in the final fibres. Scanning electron microscopy showed the fibres to have smooth cylindrical morphologies with the optimised parameters (Figure 3.2(a)).

DSC data (Figure 3.2(b)) show that the pure indomethacin powder is crystalline, because there is a large endothermic peak at 159°C which corresponds to melting. Pure PVP has a broad endotherm below around 125°C. This is not a melting event (melting endotherms are sharp peaks), but arises due to the evaporation of water: PVP is a very hygroscopic polymer, and will absorb water from the air. The fibres show no sharp melting endotherms in their DSC traces, with only very shallow endotherms below 100°C. The latter most likely occurs as a result of the fibres absorbing some water upon storage. Therefore, it can be concluded that the drug is amorphously distributed in the fibres. This should accelerate dissolution, since there will be no intermolecular interactions between indomethacin molecules.

The findings from DSC are confirmed by XRD (Figure 3.2(c)). The pattern for pure indomethacin contains many sharp peaks (Bragg reflections), because it is a crystalline material with the molecules arranged in a regular manner. In contrast, there are no sharp peaks in the patterns of either raw PVP or the drug-loaded fibres. This confirms them to be amorphous materials, with no long-range order. The XRD data thus agree well with the DSC findings.

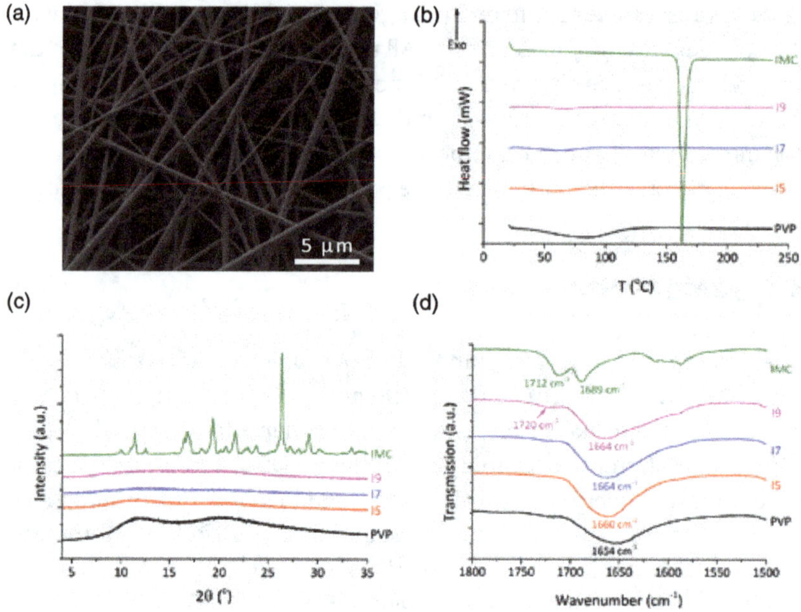

Figure 3.2 Exemplar data obtained on electrospun fibre formulations, as reported for poly(vinyl pyrrolidone) (PVP)/indomethacin systems by Lopez *et al.* (a) Scanning electron microscopy image of fibres with a 9.1% w/w drug content; (b) differential scanning calorimetry thermograms; (c) X-ray diffraction patterns; and (d) infrared spectra. IMC denotes pure indomethacin, and I5, I7 and I9 are fibres with 9.1%, 23.1% and 33.3% w/w drug loadings. (Adapted from Lopez, F. L.; Shearman, G. C.; Gaisford, S.; Williams, G. R. 'Amorphous formulations of indomethacin and griseofulvin prepared by electrospinning.' *Mol. Pharm.* 11 (2014): 4327–4338.)

Infrared spectra for the formulations are shown in Figure 3.2(d). Indomethacin shows carboxylate vibrations at 1689 and 1712 cm^{-1}, while the C=O band for PVP can be observed at 1654 cm^{-1}. In the formulations with 9.1% and 23.1% w/w drug contents, the carboxylate bands from the drug and PVP have merged into one broad band, at *ca.* 1660 or 1664 cm^{-1}. This shift in peak positions can be attributed to intermolecular interactions between the two components of the fibres.

When the drug loading was raised to 33.3% w/v, a shoulder on the main peak at 1664 cm^{-1} could be seen at 1720 cm^{-1}. The observation of this additional peak can be attributed to the increased drug content. Again, it can be seen that the position is shifted from that in the raw material, indicative of intermolecular interactions. Overall, therefore, it can be concluded that the PVP/indomethacin fibres exist as amorphous solid dispersions, stabilised by intermolecular interactions between the two constituents.

3.5 Fast-dissolving drug delivery systems

Fast-dissolving drug delivery systems (FD-DDSs) were initially developed in the late 1970s and have attracted a great deal of investment from the pharmaceutical industry.[19] Rather than releasing their drug cargo in the stomach or small intestine like most oral formulations, FD-DDSs either dissolve or disintegrate in the mouth in a few seconds. Since their drug cargo is released directly and rapidly in the mouth, where there are large numbers of blood vessels, the drug can quickly reach the systemic circulation. Thus, FD-DDSs can enhance bioavailability and give rapid onset of action.[20] This can be very beneficial for a number of situations, for instance with children or the elderly (who might struggle to swallow large tablets), or where very rapid relief of symptoms is required. Unlike tablets, which can be difficult to swallow, FD-DDSs can be applied universally without requiring any water to aid in swallowing.

3.5.1 Electrospun fast-dissolving drug delivery systems

Electrospun fibres have been widely explored as FD-DDSs. They have a number of properties which make them very suitable for this application. First, the drug is typically amorphously dispersed in the fibre, usually as an ASD. This means that there is no lattice energy barrier to dissolution, because the drug molecules are randomly arranged in the polymer matrix with no drug–drug intermolecular interactions. The presence of long-chain polymer molecules in the fibre will provide steric hindrance to any recrystallisation occurring, and thus the ASDs can have long-term stability (see section 1.3.4). If the fibres are made of a water-soluble and fast-dissolving polymer, then they will dissolve very rapidly into an aqueous medium. They are aided in this by the high surface-area-to-volume ratio of electrospun fibre mats, coupled with their high porosity; a high specific surface area accelerates dissolution, and the high porosity makes water ingress into the centre of the fibre mat easy and rapid.

One of the first reports of an electrospun FD-DDS came from Zhu's group in 2009.[21] Fibres loaded with the non-steroidal anti-inflammatory drug (NSAID) ibuprofen were prepared based on PVP with a molecular weight of 58 kDa. Using a polymer concentration of 30% w/v, fibres could be electrospun with drug loadings of 20% and 33% w/w in the dried products. The fibres had smooth cylindrical morphologies, although at the higher loading some drug particles could be seen at the fibre surface. Analysis by DSC and XRD proved the fibres to be amorphous materials, with no evidence of any crystalline drug being present. When added to water, the fibres disintegrated into small aggregates in less than 10 s, and all the drug loading was freed into solution within 1 min. Since the fibre mats had thicknesses of less than 1 mm, it was proposed that they have great potential for use as oral fast-dissolving films. The mats are also flexible, and can be easily cut into different shapes suitable for sublingual (under the tongue) or buccal (to the cheek) delivery.

PVP is a particularly useful polymer for FD-DDSs, because it is very hydrophilic and dissolves rapidly into water. A range of drug-loaded PVP fibres have thus been reported, containing active ingredients as diverse as irbesartan (used for treating high blood pressure),[22] ketoprofen (an NSAID),[23] mebeverine hydrochloride (an antispasmodic drug also used for dental analgesia),[24] vitamin D,[25] isosorbide dinitrate (used for treating angina),[26] borneol[27] (a common ingredient in traditional Chinese medicine) and curcumin[28] (a natural product thought to have a range of health benefits). In all cases, the formulations behave similarly. Fibres are produced which are largely smooth and cylindrical, and contain the drug in the amorphous form (as demonstrated by XRD and DSC). The fibre mats disintegrate very rapidly (in a few seconds) and free all their drug loading into solution in a few minutes. Exemplar data for curcumin-loaded systems[28] are given in Figure 3.3.

Other water-soluble polymers are also suitable for use in FD-DDSs, and poly(vinyl alcohol) (PVA) fibres loaded with caffeine or riboflavin have been reported by Li *et al.*[29] As previously, the drug was found to be loaded in the fibres in the amorphous physical form, and the formulations released their drug cargo very rapidly (within 4 min). The fibres were found to perform much better than analogous cast films (made by pouring the drug/polymer solution into a Petri dish and allowing the solvent to evaporate slowly), with significantly faster release from the former. This can be attributed both to the higher surface area and porosity of the fibres, and also to the rapid nature of electrospinning preventing any crystallisation of the active ingredients. Crystallisation is much more likely when cast films are made, because the solvent evaporation rate is slow and

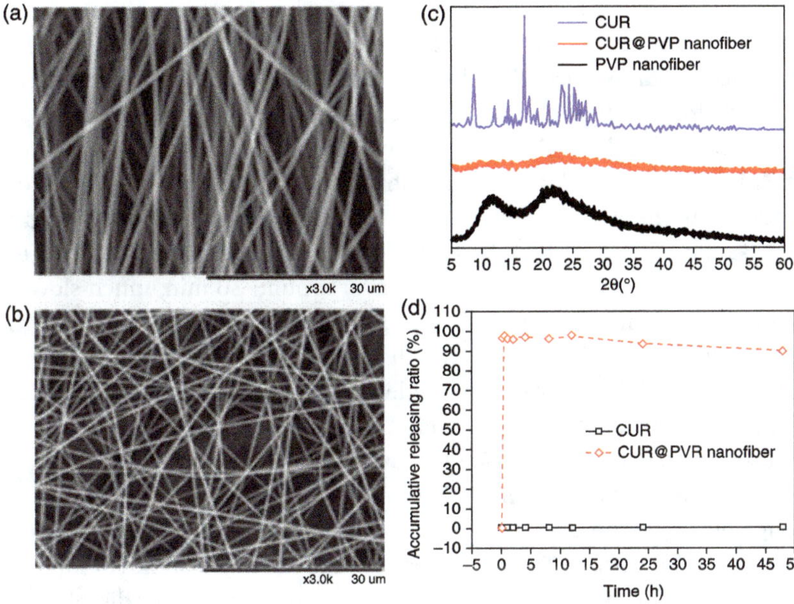

Figure 3.3 Experimental data for curcumin (CUR)-loaded poly(vinyl pyrrolidone) (PVP) fibres. Scanning electron microscopy images of (a) pure PVP and (b) PVP/curcumin fibres show them to comprise smooth cylindrical entities; (c) X-ray diffraction (XRD) shows that, while the pure drug (blue) is crystalline with many Bragg reflections in its XRD pattern, the fibres (red and black) are amorphous systems; and (d) the fibres release their drug loading much more quickly than pure curcumin dissolves. (Reproduced with permission from Wang, C.; Ma, C.; Wu, Z.; Liang, H.; Yan, P.; Song, J.; Ma, N.; Zhao, Q. 'Enhanced bioavailability and anticancer effect of curcumin-loaded electrospun nanofiber: *In vitro* and *in vivo* study.' *Nanoscale Res. Lett.* 10 (2015): 439.)

therefore there is time for molecular reorganisation to take place. PEO has also been explored for accelerating drug release, for instance for the beta-blocker carvedilol.[30]

3.5.2 Caveats

It is important to note that simply electrospinning fibres containing a drug and hydrophilic polymer will not necessarily result in the very fast release discussed here. If the drug loading is too high (above its solubility limit in the polymer) then crystallisation may occur, meaning that for at least a portion of the drug there is an energy barrier to dissolution. This has been seen by Taepaiboon *et al.* when making PVA-based fibres.[31] The presence of some crystalline drug in the fibres led to their performing similarly to cast films in terms of drug release.

The molecular weight of the polymer and the release environment are also important. For instance, Ahmad's group prepared PVP fibres loaded with the NSAID indomethacin, using PVP with a molecular weight of 1.3 million Da.[32] Although drug release was accelerated compared to the raw indomethacin, this occurred over around 30 min, much slower than the systems discussed above. This can be ascribed to the high molecular weight of PVP used, which results in its molecules being very long. There will be extensive entanglements between the PVP molecules in the fibre, which will take time to unravel. This will lead to slower dissolution than with the lower-molecular-weight PVPs used above.

In another example, Baskakova *et al.* explored PVP-based fibres for drug delivery to the eye.[33] In an *in vitro* model of the eye, release occurred over more than 100 h. This can be ascribed to the low volumes of fluid in the eye (< 5 mL, as opposed to the 1 L scale typically used for dissolution testing; see section 1.4.5.1).

3.5.3 Multicomponent formulations

It is possible to prepare systems more complex than a simple binary mixture of drug and polymer. This can be helpful to overcome some of the problems associated with oral FD-DDSs. Since the drug is released in the mouth, it is important to consider the taste (palatability) of the formulation. Many drugs are bitter-tasting, and if the formulation tastes unpleasant then there is a risk a patient will not take the required medication.

In one approach to solve this issue, Samprasit *et al.* reported three-component fibres made of PVP, meloxicam (an NSAID) and a cyclodextrin (CD).[34] CDs are cup-like molecules with a hydrophilic exterior and hydrophobic interior. They can encapsulate hydrophobic molecules in their interior, thus hiding them from an external aqueous environment. CDs might hence be used to improve the solubility and mask the taste of hydrophobic active ingredients. Additional fibre formulations were prepared containing menthol and aspartate as taste-masking agents. While the CD alone was not sufficient to hide the bitter taste of meloxicam in palatability studies, the addition of menthol and aspartate was able to do so effectively.

Fibres may also be prepared containing combinations of drugs. For instance, Illangakoon *et al.* produced fibres of PVP loaded with paracetamol and caffeine (often used together to treat colds and influenza).[19c]

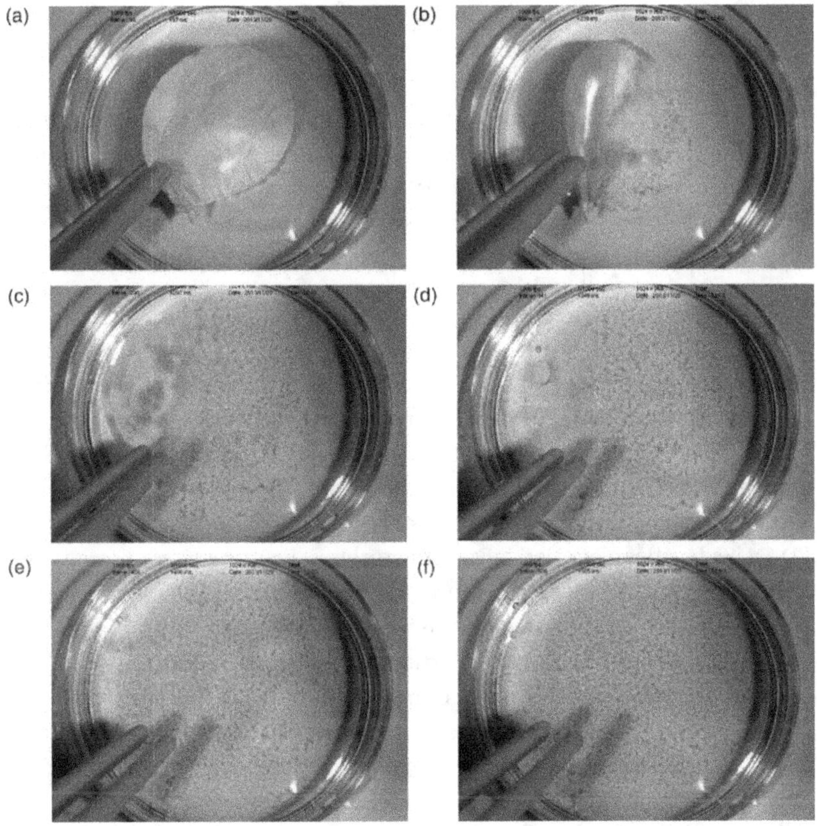

Figure 3.4 Images taken with a high-speed camera depicting the rapid disintegration of paracetamol/caffeine-loaded poly(vinyl pyrrolidone) (PVP) fibres prepared by Illangakoon *et al.* Stills from a video are given (a) 0; (b) 133; (c) 200; (d) 243; (e) 303; and (f) 408 ms after the fibres were added to a Petri dish containing simulated saliva. (Reproduced with permission from Illangakoon, U. E.; Gill, H.; Shearman, G. C.; Parhizkar, M.; Mahalingam, S.; Chatterton, N. P.; Williams, G. R. 'Fast dissolving paracetamol/caffeine nanofibers prepared by electrospinning.' *Int. J. Pharm.* 477 (2014): 369–379. Copyright Elsevier 2014.[19c])

The fibre mats disintegrated within 300 ms (Figure 3.4), and both drugs were fully released within 200 s. A raspberry flavouring was also incorporated into the fibres to help with taste masking. Vrbata *et al.* have similarly reported fibres containing both sumatriptan succinate and naproxen, which might be used as oral FD-DDSs to treat migranes.[35]

More complex systems can also be generated containing multiple excipients. One example of this comes from Yu *et al.*[36] PVP fibres were prepared loaded with the antioxidant ferulic acid (FA), sodium dodecyl sulfate and sucralose. Sucralose was added to mask the taste of the very bitter FA. Sodium dodecyl sulfate acts as a permeation enhancer, aiding the drug to pass through the mucosa in the mouth to reach the systemic circulation. The fibres could increase the FA permeation rate by more than 13-fold.

3.5.4 Stability

The stability of ASDs is a major concern for the pharmaceutical industry, because of the propensity for an amorphous system to convert to a crystalline material over time. It is vitally important that the medicine taken by a patient has the intended performance. This might well not be the case if there is recrystallisation during storage. The stability of electrospun FD-DDSs has been studied by several authors. Brettmann *et al.* prepared indomethacin/PVP fibres and found that they remained amorphous after being stored for 6 months in a desiccator at 40°C.[37] Illangakoon and co-workers determined that PVP fibres containing mebeverine hydrochloride remained as ASDs over 12 months' storage in a desiccator.[24]

Lopez and colleagues investigated in detail long-term stability for PVP-based fibres loaded with either indomethacin or griseofulvin (an antifungal agent).[18] These active ingredients were chosen because of their very different glass-forming behaviour. Indomethacin can be made amorphous very easily and forms stable glasses, but amorphous griseofulvin is known to convert rapidly to the crystalline state. Both drugs could be converted into ASDs with PVP, even with drug loadings of up to 33%. Drug release from all the composites was very rapid (< 10 min). In stability studies, there was some evidence for phase separation of the active ingredient and polymer after 8 months of storage in a desiccator, but no crystallisation was observed and the fibres remained amorphous after this time.

Nagy's team have also looked in detail at stability, in their case for poly(vinylpyrrolidone/vinyl acetate) (PVPVA) FD-DDSs loaded with itraconazole.[38] The amorphous form was preserved over 1 year at 25°C and 60% relative humidity (RH), but at 40°C and 75% RH some recrystallisation was observed over 3 months.

Overall, it appears that electrospun ASDs can retain their stability for a prolonged period of time. However, the hydroscopic nature of the polymers used for such systems can lead to recystallisation at high humidities, since the fibres will be able to absorb moisture. This will enhance molecular mobility, allowing the drug molecules to reorient themselves into regular arrangements and form crystals. Packaging the formulations under nitrogen should prevent this instability from arising, however, and is an eminently affordable option for industry (crisps are packaged under nitrogen to keep them fresh).

3.6 Extended-release systems

The United States Pharmacopoeia (USP) defines a modified-release dosage form as one where 'the drug release characteristics of time course and/or location are chosen to accomplish therapeutic or convenience objectives not offered by conventional dosage forms such as solutions, ointments, or promptly dissolving dosage forms'.[39] Extended-release systems (also known as controlled-release, prolonged-release, or sustained or slow-release) free their drug cargo over a prolonged period of time in the body. This can be beneficial to avoid there being an excessively high drug loading in the systemic circulation, or for drugs which can be degraded in the blood. To achieve extended release with electrospun fibres, a polymer is chosen which dissolves or degrades slowly, or one which is insoluble. As for the FD-DDSs, it is usual that the fibres comprise ASDs, with the drug amorphously distributed in the fibres, but because the polymer itself is slow to dissolve or does not dissolve at all, drug release should be delayed.

Extended-release fibres may be prepared from non-biodegradable or biodegradable polymers.[40] The former do not degrade in the body, while the latter are broken down into small components over time. Biodegradable polyesters such as PCL, poly(glycolic acid) (PGA), PLA and PLGA have been widely studied.[40] Suitable choices of non-degradable polymers might be polyurethane, polycarbonate or nylon-6. Naturally occurring biopolymers (e.g. silk, collagen, chitosan, gelatin or alginate) are also appropriate. However, biopolymers are usually extracted from natural sources and invariably have batch-to-batch variations in molecular weight, purity, distribution of charged groups and crystallinity. This material inconsistency makes it difficult to generate reproducible electrospun products from different batches of material, and complicates practical applications.[41] In addition, owing to their strong inter- and intramolecular forces, many biopolymers only dissolve in a limited number of solvents that are unsuitable for electrospinning (e.g. polysaccharides such as cellulose and chitin, proteins such as collagen).

They may also form an ionic solution; when such solutions are electrified, the ionic groups generate high repulsive forces, disrupting continuous fibre formation and leading to defects (e.g. with chitosan and gelatin). Biopolymers are thus often mixed with a secondary polymer such as PEO or PVA to facilitate the electrospinning process.

3.6.1 Applications

Kenawy was the first to report an extended-release electrospun fibre system.[1] PLA, PEVA and blend fibres were prepared loaded with the antibiotic tetracycline hydrochloride, and as a result release could be extended over more than 120 h. Such systems have a range of applications, most likely in the form of wound dressings or implantable formulations. One obvious indication in which they might be used is the treatment of cancer, and a number of studies have been reported looking at electrospun fibres in this regard. PLGA fibres loaded with the anticancer drug paclitaxel have been shown to give release extended over 60 days, and to inhibit the proliferation of glioma cancer cells effectively.[42] Fibres made from a mixture of PLGA and PLA and loaded with cisplatin, another anticancer drug, also show promise for cancer treatments, with drug release occurring over at least 30 days, and reductions in cancer cell viability.[43] In addition, the inclusion of targeting molecules in the fibres can help target drug delivery to particular cell types; for instance, folic acid has been incorporated into fibres specifically to deliver viral vectors to cancer cells, while normal cells are unaffected.[44]

Other applications of extended-release fibres include in regenerative medicine. Puppi *et al.* electrospun PLGA fibres containing retinoic acid, with the aim of making scaffolds for tissue regeneration.[45] Their materials were seen to retain their morphology over 12 weeks, with continuous drug release during this time. Cells were able to proliferate on the fibre mats. PCL fibres loaded with heparin have been reported to release around 50% of their drug loading over 14 days, and to have potential for delivering heparin to the site of vascular injury to prevent stenosis (narrowing of the arteries).[46] More details on tissue-engineering applications are given in section 3.12.

The prevention of infection in wounds or after surgery is another area to have attracted attention. For instance, PCL fibres with potential applications in hernia repair have been produced containing antibiotics or antibacterial agents.[47] Zhang *et al.* made blends of PLGA and poly(dioxanone) (PDO), poly(ethylene glycol)-*b*-poly(D,L-lactide-*co*-glycolide) (PELA) or PGA loaded with ciprofloxacin hydrochloride, moxifloxacin or moxifloxicin

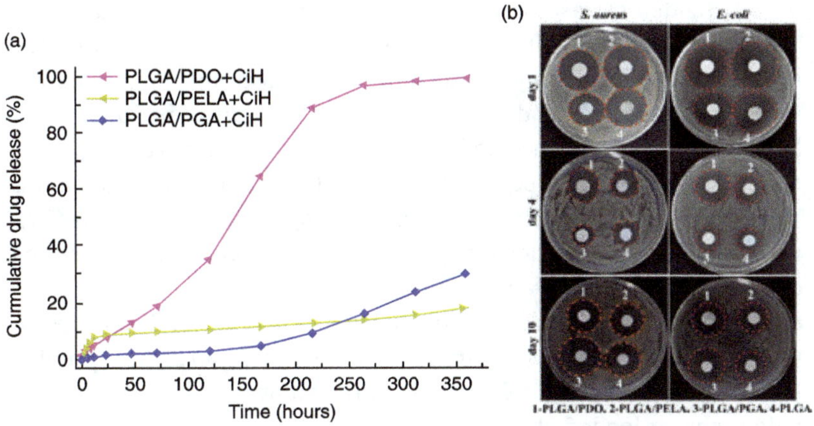

Figure 3.5 Data obtained by Zhang *et al.* for poly(lactic-co-glycolic acid) (PLGA) blend fibres loaded with ciprofloxacin hydrochloride (CiH). (a) Variation in the blend of polymers used leads to distinctly different release properties, with drug release occurring over more than 200 h in some cases. (b) The CiH-loaded fibres are able to inhibit bacterial growth effectively over at least 10 days. PDO: poly(dioxanone); PELA: poly(ethylene glycol)-*b*-poly(D,L-lactide-co-glycolide); PGA: poly(glycolic acid). (Reproduced with permission from Zhang, Z.; Tang, J.; Wang, H.; Xia, Q.; Xu, S.; Han, C. C. 'Controlled antibiotics release system through simple blended electrospun fibers for sustained antibacterial effects.' *ACS Appl. Mater. Interfaces* 7 (2015): 26400–26404. Copyright American Chemical Society 2015.)

hydrochloride.[48] Selected data from this work are shown in Figure 3.5. The blend of polymers used permits control to be exercised on the release pattern, with some formulations able to give approximately linear drug release over more than 200 h. The fibres could also effectively inhibit bacterial growth *in vitro*.[48] These systems might effectively be used as an implant to prevent infection after abdominal surgery.

Other researchers have looked at wound healing. PCL and PLA fibres containing a vitamin D_3 derivative have been electrospun and found to free their drug cargo over around 10–15 days, potentially suitable for wound healing.[49] Polyvinylidene fluoride fibres have also been explored in this setting, and release of the active ingredient observed over 45–90 h.[50] In other work, Zamani and co-workers explored metronidazole benzoate-loaded PCL fibres for periodontal diseases (inflammation and degeneration of the gums).[51] Drug release was prolonged over 20 days.

Extended release over shorter time periods than those discussed above can also be useful. For instance, it takes approximately 1 day for a formulation taken orally to pass through the gastrointestinal tract, and so a system able to extend release over the 10–20-h time period could be beneficial for making once-daily medicines. Transdermal (through skin) delivery over this time period would also lead to potent formulations. Yu *et al.* have performed work in which poly(acrylonitrile) (PAN) fibres were loaded with acyclovir and explored as a potential transdermal drug delivery system.[52] As for the fibres discussed above, the drug was amorphously distributed in the polymer matrix at lower loadings (10% w/w), but at higher drug concentrations (up to 20% w/w) some crystalline material was observed. Release was sustained over 12 h. In other work, indomethacin-loaded fibres prepared from EC and zein (water-insoluble polymers) have been found to extend drug release over more than 20 h.[53] This type of system might thus be useful for oral administration.

Vaginal applications have also been proposed for extended-release electrospun fibres, as reviewed by Blakney *et al.*[3b]

3.6.2 Drawbacks and release mechanisms

One key drawback encountered with using monolithic fibres from monoaxial spinning for extended release is that, in the majority of cases, there is a burst of release at the start of the process. This is because of the fibre mat's very high surface-area-to-volume ratio, which results in a significant proportion of the drug molecules in the fibres being near to the surface. These can rapidly diffuse out into solution, even if the polymer matrix is slow-dissolving or insoluble. The burst is not a problem in the context of FD-DDSs where all the active ingredient is released very quickly, but with an extended-release formulation the rate of release (and thus the amount of drug reaching the bloodstream) will be much quicker immediately after the medicine has been taken than later on.

The burst release effect can be minimised with a low drug loading, but for clinical applications high doses (10–100 mg of drug per dose) are often required. These necessitate high drug loadings in the fibres, and present additional challenges for sustaining drug release. Higher drug loadings lead to larger amounts of the active ingredient at or near the surface. Many studies have been performed with low loadings (< 1% w/w), and thus the formulations prepared have limited clinical applications. For instance, Ball *et al.*[3a] made fibres from biodegradable polymers and explored them for extended release, with antibacterial applications in mind. Maraviroc, azidothymidine, acyclovir and glycerylmonolaurate-loaded fibres were generated successfully, and the formulations were found to be non-toxic. Although the fibres provided sustained release in some cases, the drug loading was only 1% w/w, and so the formulations as they stand cannot directly be translated to the clinic.[3a]

If the burst release is a major problem for a particular system, there are several possible solutions. One is coaxial or multi-axial electrospinning, as will be discussed in Chapter 4. Another option is to bond the active ingredient of interest covalently to the polymer and then spin this into fibres, a concept demonstrated by Jalvandi and co-workers in the case of levofloxacin and chitosan.[54]

Natu *et al.* have investigated the effect of drug location and physical form on the release rate from fibres electrospun from slow-dissolving polymers, using acetazolamide and timolol maleate as hydrophobic and hydrophilic model drugs, respectively.[55] At low concentrations (below the drug solubility in the polymer: 1.16–1.55% w/w for acetazolamide; 0.86–0.88% w/w for timolol), the drug was amorphously distributed in the fibres, but crystalline material was observed when the drug content was greater than its solubility in the polymer. With the low concentrations, where the drug was well encapsulated in the fibres, there was only a small initial burst of release. However, at high concentrations (above the drug solubility in the polymer: 12.67% w/w for acetazolamide; 6.99–7.6% w/w for timolol) this burst was much greater, attributed to the presence of crystalline drug particles at the edge of the fibres.

The mechanism of drug release from extended-release fibres can be controlled by one or more of three processes: drug diffusion through the polymer, polymer degradation and drug dissolution into solution.[2a] This makes the details of the release process complex, and it can be difficult to predict how a particular system will behave. It would be intuitively expected that if drug release is controlled solely by the diffusion of the drug through the polymer, then larger-diameter fibres will release more slowly because there will be a longer path through which the drug must diffuse to reach solution. However, this is not always the case, and the diffusion distance is not the only factor which changes with fibre diameter. Verreck *et al.*[56] posited that smaller-diameter fibres might be more tightly packed, inhibiting the swelling of the fibre matrix and the ingress of water. Fibre diameter is typically controlled through formulation properties such as polymer concentration and solvent choice, but these can also affect the dispersion of drug in the fibre products (among other factors), which must be considered when developing monolithic extended-release fibres.[2a]

There are several reports in the literature confirming the importance of considering formulations on a case-by-case basis. Studies performed with PLA (molecular weight = 75–120 kDa) as the polymer matrix found that the rate of drug delivery for tetracycline became slower as the fibre diameter increased from 220 ± 60 nm to 360 ± 70 nm, and to 830 ± 280 nm.[57] However, when the fibres were loaded with chlorotetracycline the release rate became faster with an increase in fibre diameter from 200 nm to 1.6 μm. The opposite release behaviours were thought to be because multiple factors, including the fibres' swelling behaviour and the drug's solubility in the polymer matrix and the release medium, influenced the release profile.[57]

A wide variety of active ingredients can be mixed with a polymer and electrospun into fibres, as has been described above. However, most examples of drug release extending beyond seven days relate to macromolecules or hydrophobic small-molecule drugs.[58] These active ingredients have at least one of the following characteristics: poor solubility in aqueous media, large molecular size and/or favourable intermolecular interactions with the hydrophobic polymers typically used for extended-release formulations. All these characteristics help to retard the rate at which the drugs are freed from the polymer matrix. In contrast, hydrophilic small-molecule drugs are very difficult to formulate for extended release because they have high solubility in the release medium, and more favourable interactions with an aqueous environment than with the polymer in the fibres. These factors promote drug release from the fibres.

3.7 pH-controlled delivery

3.7.1 Oral administration

When a medicine is given orally, the variations in pH occurring in the intestinal tract offer the potential to provide delayed release. The pH of the stomach is acidic, typically at around 1–2, while that of the small intestine is close to neutral (with variations depending on the exact location). Thus, if a fibre is made of a pH-sensitive polymer, which is insoluble at low pH but soluble at neutral pH, then it might be expected that its drug loading would be released only in the small intestine. This is potentially very useful, because there are many drugs (such as the NSAIDs) which can cause serious irritation to the stomach, and others which are degraded by the acid or enzymes present.

A number of researchers have explored these possibilities. In 2007, Wang *et al.* produced erythromycin-loaded fibres made of hydroxypropylmethylcellulose phthalate (HPMCP).[59] Erythromycin (an antibiotic) is rendered inactive at low pH, and thus it is desirable to prevent it dissolving in the stomach. Since HPMCP is insoluble below pH 5.5, it was reasoned that fibres made of this polymer could have potential here. As expected, drug release was much slower at pH 1.2 than at 6.8.

The Eudragit polymers, a family of materials based on methacrylates, have also received extensive attention for electrospun pH-sensitive drug delivery systems. For instance, Eudragit L100-55 dissolves at pH 5.5, L100 at pH 6.0 and S100 at 7.0; below these pH values, the polymers are insoluble. Thus, targeting to the small intestine should be possible. The polymers can be successfully processed by electrospinning, with Shen *et al.* reporting Eudragit L100-55 fibres loaded with diclofenac sodium in 2011.[60] The formulations were subject to a dissolution test where the fibres were first placed in a pH 1.0 solution (to mimic the stomach) and then transferred to a pH 6.8 buffer (representative of the small intestine). Less than 3% of the diclofenac content was released at pH 1.0, while at pH 6.8 extended release over up to 5 h was observed. These findings suggested that the fibres have potential for targeting release to the small intestine. Similar results have been found by Akhgari and co-workers for indomethacin-loaded fibres.[61]

The work of Shen and Akhgari used an acidic drug (one which can be ionised through loss of a proton). Such active ingredients have solubility which increases with pH, and thus will always have a lesser tendency to be released from a formulation at low pH than under neutral conditions. Illangakoon *et al.* prepared Eudragit L100-55 fibres containing the basic drug mebeverine hydrochloride.[24] This will be more soluble at low pH, and thus one might expect a greater amount of release in conditions representative of the stomach than with an acidic drug. Smooth cylindrical fibres were obtained with drug loadings of 30% w/w or below, but when the loading was increased to 55% w/w the fibres were observed to break apart upon storage (Figure 3.6(a) and (b)). As for the FD-DDS materials discussed previously, the fibres comprise ASDs with no evidence for any crystalline drug being present.

After 2 h at pH 2 some 15–25% of the mebeverine loading had been freed into solution, as would be expected given the basic nature of mebeverine. However, the fibres release much less drug at this pH than a Eudragit/mebeverine physical mixture. At pH 6.8, extended release over *ca.* 8 hours was observed. Thus, using Eudragit-based fibres can be a suitable route to prepare delayed-release oral formulations even for basic drugs. However, it should be noted that the same burst release issue as

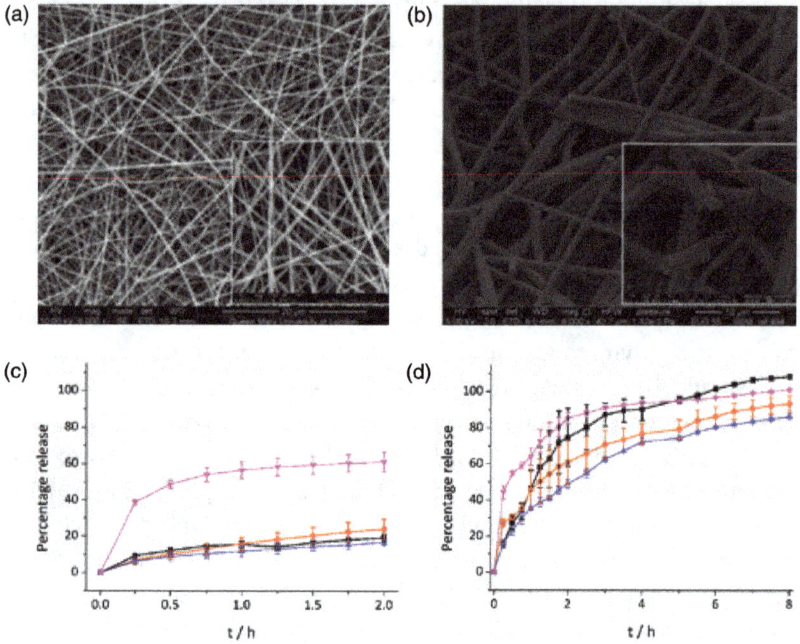

Figure 3.6 Experimental data on mebeverine chloride-loaded Eudragit fibres prepared by electrospinning. Scanning electron microscopy images of the fibres with (a) 30% and (b) 55% w/w drug contents; (c) drug release at pH 2; and (d) the release profiles obtained at pH 6.8. Release data are shown for fibres containing 5 (■), 15 (●) and 30 (▲) % w/w mebeverine hydrochloride contents, together with a physical mixture of drug and Eudragit as a control (▼). (Reproduced with permission from Illangakoon, U. E.; Nazir, T.; Williams, G. R.; Chatterton, N. P. 'Mebeverine-loaded electrospun nanofibers: Physicochemical characterization and dissolution studies.' *J. Pharm. Sci.* 103 (2014): 283–292. Copyright Elsevier 2014.)

described in section 3.6.2 arises with these monolithic fibre systems. Further, some authors have observed significant amounts of release at low pH even with an acidic drug. Karthikeyan *et al.* reported fibres made from a blend of zein (a water-insoluble polymer) and Eudragit S100, loaded with aceclofenac (an acidic NSAID) and pantaprazole (a basic drug used to help prevent side effects when patients are taking NSAIDs for extended time periods).[62] While the fibres were able to prevent pantaprazole release effectively at pH 1, some 25% of the aceclofenac was freed into solution at this pH. This may be a result of the way in which the fibres were prepared from a mixture of pantaprazole/Eudragit and aceclofenac/zein solutions, but nevertheless shows that simple monolithic fibres are not always effective for pH-targeted release.

3.7.2 Anticancer applications

Another route to impart pH sensitivity on electrospun fibres is to incorporate a pH-sensitive agent other than the polymer. Cui's group were able to prepare poly(L-lactic acid) fibres which released their drug cargo faster at lower pHs by the simple expedient of including sodium bicarbonate in the formulation.[63] The fibres contained 5-fluorouracil (5-FU), an anticancer drug, and were found to be able to inhibit the growth of human osteosarcoma cancer cells while being harmless to fibroblast cells. This is because the tumour microenvironment is somewhat more acidic than normal physiological pH. At pH 5.0, sodium bicarbonate will react with the protons present, forming carbon dioxide gas. As the gas leaves the fibres, it creates channels in them. These channels make it easier for water to enter the fibres to dissolve the drug, and for the drug to diffuse into solution. Thus, in this particular instance 5-FU is freed more rapidly in the slightly acidic pH conditions of the cancer environment, and cancer cell proliferation is inhibited over a 4-day *in vitro* culture. At the normal physiological pH (7.4), the sodium bicarbonate in the fibres does not react, and thus no pores are created and drug release is slower. Similar results have been reported for ibuprofen-loaded PLGA fibres containing sodium bicarbonate.[64]

Interactions between the drug and polymer may also be used to provide pH sensitivity, if these change with pH. Salehi *et al.* have reported such a system built on poly(*N*-isopropylacrylamide-co-methacrylic acid-co-vinylpyrrolidone) and the anticancer drug doxorubicin.[65] At pH 7.4, the polymer is ionised and favourable electrostatic interactions with the drug cause release to be slowed. At pH 5.4, representative of the cancer microenvironment, the polymer is uncharged, and thus these interactions are reduced and the drug releases more rapidly.

3.8 Pulsatile release

Pulsatile release refers to an on/off pattern of release, with bursts of release separated by periods where no further drug is freed from a formulation. This can be particularly beneficial for conditions which follow the body's natural circadian rhythms and are worse at particular times of day. Asthma attacks are more common late at night, for instance, while rheumatoid arthritis is worse in the morning. Electrospun fibres have not been much explored for pulsatile release, but there is one report of this modality being achieved.

Kaassis and co-workers made fibres from PEO, sodium alginate (a naturally occurring polysaccharide which is insoluble at low pH but freely soluble at pHs higher than around 5) and sodium ibuprofen.[66] While the other fibre systems discussed in this chapter are obtained as flat mats, in this study the fibres were found to form a 'mountain' shape growing up from the collector (Figure 3.7(a)). Evidence for crystalline sodium ibuprofen was found in XRD and DSC. At pH 6.8 (representative of the small intestine), the fibres free their drug loading within around 20 min (Figure 3.7(b)). However, at pH 3 (representative of the stomach in the fed state) clear pulsatile release is seen (Figure 3.7(c)), with two stages of release and a lag between them. The percentage of drug in the first stage can be controlled through the ibuprofen content of the fibres (Figure 3.7(c)), while the lag between them can be varied by altering the amount of alginate present (Figure 3.7(d)).

3.9 Multilayer materials

As discussed above, through variation of the polymer used to prepare electrospun fibres, it is possible to provide a range of drug delivery patterns. It is also possible to produce a mat made of multiple layers of monolithic fibres, with each layer made of a different material, to provide more complex release profiles. Blagbrough's team have used this approach extensively to prepare multilayer meshes for wound-healing purposes.

In the first such study, Alhusein *et al.* used solutions of either PCL or PEVA.[67] By sequentially electrospinning layers of each polymer on to the collector, they could produce a three-layered formulation with alternating PCL/PEVA/PCL layers. The antibiotic tetracycline hydrochloride was either incorporated into all three layers, or just in the central PEVA layer. Simple two-component fibre mats of PCL/tetracycline and PEVA/tetracycline were also prepared. While the PCL/tetracycline formulation released all its drug within 1 day, the PEVA/tetracycline fibres were able to extend this over 8 days. The three-layer PCL/PEVA/PCL system could extend tetracycline release over 14 days; when the drug was present in all three layers, a burst of 60% release was seen in the early stages of the experiment, but incorporating the drug only in the central layer reduced this to 10%, and permitted

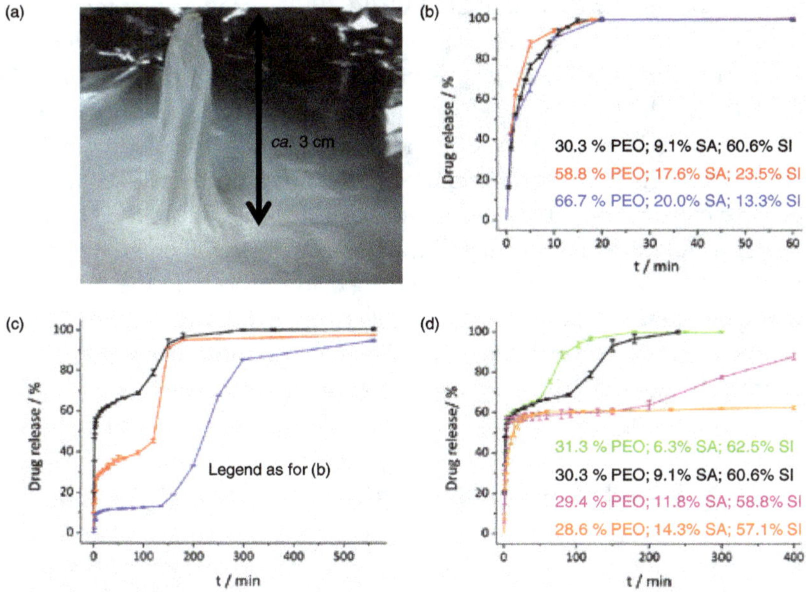

Figure 3.7 Pulsatile release from electrospun fibres comprising poly(ethylene oxide) (PEO), sodium alginate (SA) and sodium ibuprofen (SI), as reported by Kaassis *et al.*[66] (a) The mountain of fibres which was observed to form on the collector; (b) at pH 6.8 the fibres free their drug loading within 15 min; (c) at pH 3 pulsatile release is observed, with the amount of release in the first stage dictated by the ibuprofen content of the fibres; and (d) the lag between the two phases of release can be tuned by varying the sodium alginate content of the fibres. (Reproduced with permission from Kaassis, A. Y. A.; Young, N.; Sano, N.; Merchant, H. A.; Yu, D.-G.; Chatterton, N. P.; Williams, G. R. 'Pulsatile drug release from electrospun poly(ethylene oxide)–sodium alginate blend nanofibres.' *J. Mater. Chem. B* 2 (2014): 1400–1407. Copyright Royal Society of Chemistry 2014.)

an almost constant (zero-order) rate of release to be achieved. The PCL/PEVA/PCL system could also effectively inhibit bacterial growth.[68] Similar results were reported using three-layer systems with tetracycline solely in the central layer when these were fabricated from zein or zein/PCL blends.[69] The latter have been found to be potent in preventing biofilm formation, and to be compatible with human skin cells.[70]

This idea of depositing multiple fibre layers was also explored by Huang *et al.*[71] Using ketoprofen as a model drug, polymer/drug solutions were prepared using PVP and EC. PVP/EC/PVP three-layer systems were produced, with ketoprofen present in each layer. Systems were generated with the different layers having varying thickness by varying the duration of time for which each was electrospun. The products comprised ASDs, and the three-layer system was found to give a two-phase (*biphasic*) drug release pattern. The PVP layers provided a burst of release at the start of the experiment, and then extended release ensued from the EC layer. Such formulations could be beneficial because the initial burst provides a *loading dose*, rapidly increasing the drug concentration in the plasma to therapeutic levels; the second, slow-release phase can then maintain the concentration in the effective range. Huang and colleagues were able to control the extent of the burst by varying the layer thickness.[71]

3.10 Thermoresponsive systems

A number of polymers are *thermosensitive*; that is, they change properties in response to temperature variation. Such polymers have been explored in electrospinning, with most attention paid to poly(*N*-isopropyl acrylamide) (PNIPAAm). This polymer is hydrophilic at room temperature, and can dissolve in water. However, at around 32°C it undergoes a chain-to-globule transition and becomes hydrophobic. The temperature at which this arises is known as the *lower critical solution temperature* (LCST). Although PNIPAAm can be electrospun alone,[72] it is more usually blended with carrier polymers such as PEO to facilitate the spinning process.[73] The thermosensitive properties of PNIPAAm are preserved after spinning, meaning that the fibres generated change their hydrophilicity in response to temperature.

Thermosensitive fibres have attracted some attention for drug delivery purposes. Fibres made from a blend of PNIPAAm and poly(2-acrylamido-2-methylpropanesulfonic acid) release a nifedipine cargo more rapidly below the LCST than above.[74] PNIPAAm/PEO blend fibres containing vitamin B_{12} behave similarly,[75] as do PNIPAAm/EC formulations.[76] Although the exact behaviour can be tuned by varying the composition of the fibres, the *in vivo* applications of these particular formulations are not clear: a system able to control release in response to small variations in body temperature would be useful, but PNIPAAm cannot deliver this because its LCST is well below the physiological temperature range.

Where systems based on LCST polymers might be very useful, however, is in the treatment of wounds. When a wound dressing is changed, it is common for some tissue to be pulled away from the wound: this results in what are known as secondary injuries. Thermosensitive materials can be used to control cell adhesion, because interactions between cells and the polymer are much stronger above the LCST than below it. Thus, a thermosensitive wound dressing could be very beneficial if the LCST was a little below body temperature. A local low-temperature treatment would drop the temperature of the skin below the LCST, reduce the strength of interactions between the dressing and the cells around the wound, and hence prevent secondary injuries when the dressing is removed. Electrospun fibres have many properties making them suitable for wound dressings, since their high porosity allows them to absorb any fluids exuded from the wound, and their web structure helps to facilitate cell growth.

Thermoresponsive electrospun wound dressings have recently been reported by Li *et al.* using either PNIPAAm[77] or poly(di(ethylene glycol) methyl ether methacrylate)[78] as the thermosensitive polymer in a blend with poly(L-lactic acid-co-ε-caprolactone) (PLCL). The anti-bacterial drug ciprofloxacin was incorporated into the fibres to prevent infection. Ciprofloxacin was freed from the fibres over more than 200 h, and the formulations could effectively prevent bacterial growth. The thermosensitive mats were able to accelerate wound healing over fibres prepared from PLCL and ciprofloxacin alone (Figure 3.8).

3.11 Emulsion and suspension electrospinning

The above discussion has focused on electrospinning a solution of a drug and polymer. In addition, it is possible to process emulsions and suspensions, and the resultant fibres can have a number of beneficial properties.

3.11.1 Emulsions

A range of fibres have been prepared using monoaxial emulsion electrospinning. For instance, Jing's group made a water-in-oil emulsion stabilised with the surfactant sodium dodecyl sulfate.[79] The hydrophilic active pharmaceutical ingredient (API) doxorubicin hydrochloride was present in the water phase. A block copolymer (poly(ethylene glycol)-poly(L-lactic acid)) dissolved in chloroform was used to form the fibres. This copolymer is amphiphilic and has both hydrophobic and hydrophilic sections, which means that it should be able to interact with both

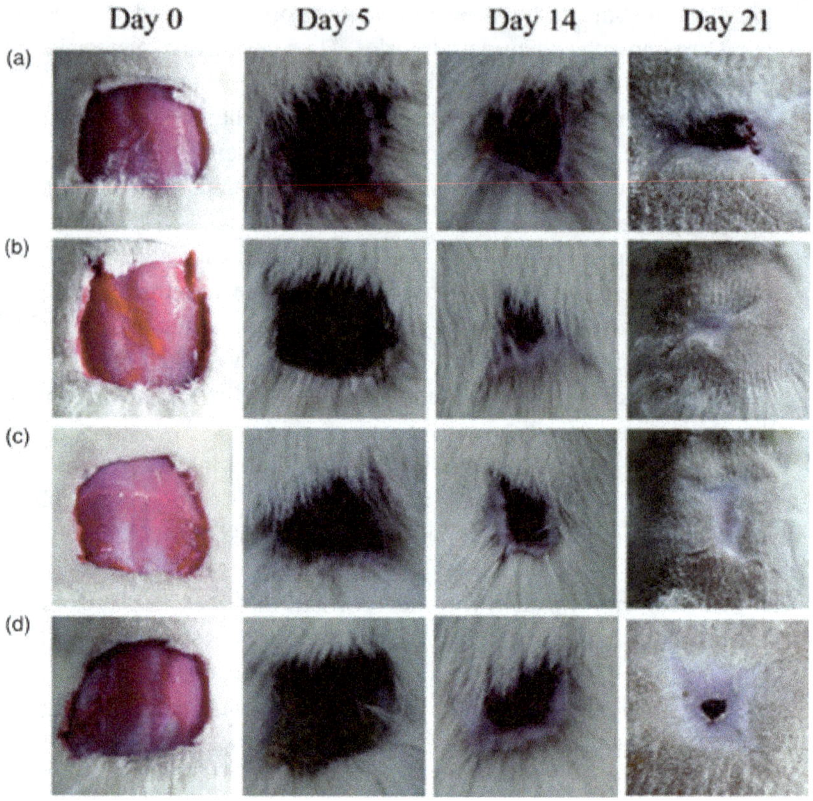

Figure 3.8 Images showing the healing of wounds inflicted on rats and treated with electrospun dressings. The wounds were treated with (a) a commercial gauze; (b) poly(*N*-isopropyl acrylamide) (PNIPAAm)/poly(L-lactide-co-ε-caprolactone) (PLCL)/ciprofloxacin fibres with a 1:1 mass ratio of the polymers; (c) PNIPAAm/PLCL/ciprofloxacin fibres with polymer mass ratio 1:2; and (d) PLCL/ciprofloxacin fibres. It is clear that the formulations containing PNIPAAm lead to faster wound healing. (Reproduced with permission from Li, H.; Williams, G. R.; Wu, J.; Wang, H.; Sun, X.; Zhu, L. M. 'Poly(N-isopropylacrylamide)/poly(l-lactic acid-co-caprolactone) fibers loaded with ciprofloxacin as wound dressing materials.' *Mater. Sci. Eng. C* 79 (2017): 245–254.[77] Copyright Elsevier 2017.)

parts of the emulsion. After electrospinning, the fibres were found to have an aqueous core/hydrophobic shell structure, despite having been produced from a monoaxial process. This was attributed to a separation of the hydrophobic and hydrophilic components of the fibres, with the surfactant at the interface. This spontaneous self-assembly of core/shell

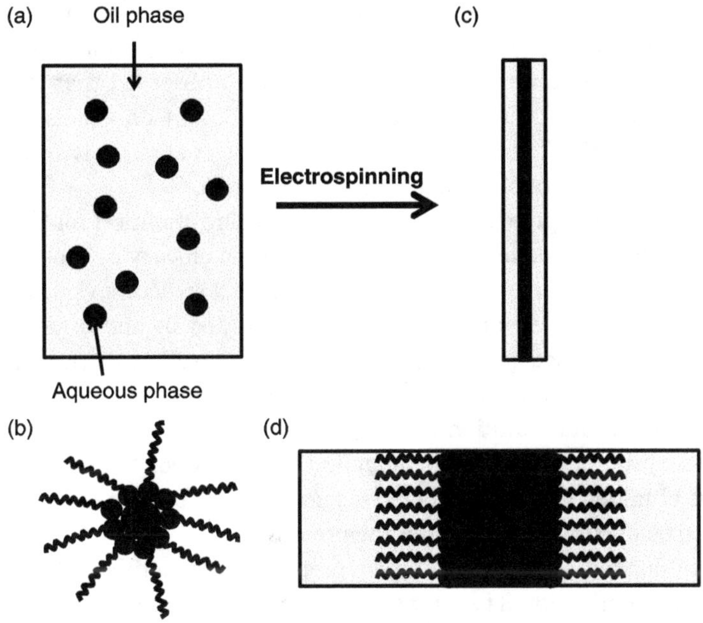

Figure 3.9 Schematic showing how a core/shell fibre can be generated from emulsion electrospinning. (a) A water-in-oil emulsion, with droplets of water dispersed throughout a continuous oil phase; (b) a close-up of a single water droplet, showing how a surfactant (an amphiphilic molecule with a hydrophilic head and hydrophobic tail) is used to stabilise the emulsion. Surfactant molecules will be arranged around the edge of the water droplets, with their hydrophilic head groups touching the droplet and their hydrophobic tails dangling into the oil phase. (c) After electrospinning a core shell fibre is formed, with (d) the surfactant molecules collected along the oil/water interface to minimise unfavourable interactions.

structures is very commonly seen in emulsion spinning. The mechanism underlying this is illustrated in Figure 3.9, and has been discussed in detail by Wang and Wang.[80]

The presence of a water-soluble active ingredient in the core of fibres spun from water-in-oil emulsions has the benefit of ameliorating any initial burst release. This was shown for the model drugs cefradine and 5-FU: fibres prepared from emulsion spinning had reduced initial burst release and a slower release rate than analogous fibres made by standard monoaxial solution spinning.[81] A lack of burst release from emulsion spun fibres was also noted with doxorubicin hydrochloride by Xu *et al.*[79]

Further, emulsion electrospinning has been demonstrated to modulate fibre properties, for instance reducing the fibre diameters in comparison with monoaxial solution electrospinning.[82] Sy *et al.* observed that the mixing of phases of different rheological properties in an emulsion caused electrospinning to occur at a much lower range of liquid viscosity than that for a conventional monoaxial solution system.[82]

The emulsion approach has attracted particular attention for the production of protein-loaded fibres. The therapeutic efficacy of protein drugs is highly dependent on their three-dimensional structure (known as the tertiary structure), and this is easily degraded by the organic solvents commonly used for electrospinning. Incorporating them into water droplets in an organic continuous phase could be an effective route to prevent protein denaturation and degradation.[83] This was reported for the model protein bovine serum albumin (BSA) in 2008.[84] Core/shell fibres were obtained via emulsion electrospinning, and protein stability appeared to be preserved throughout the process.

Protein-loaded core/shell fibres prepared through emulsion spinning have been explored for a range of applications. These include the delivery of growth factors to encourage tissue regeneration. For instance, PLCL fibres containing vascular endothelial growth factor have been shown to have potential for cardiac regeneration.[85] Vascular endothelial growth factor was released over more than 28 days, and human bone marrow-derived mesenchymal stem cells could proliferate on the fibres over a 20-day culture period. Emulsion fibres carrying a protein payload have further been investigated in bone tissue engineering, *inter alia*.[86]

Another benefit of emulsion spinning is in incorporating APIs of opposing polarity to the polymer used. As discussed in section 3.2.4, if a hydrophobic drug is loaded in a hydrophilic polymer (or vice versa) there is a risk of phase separation occurring on storage. This can be a problem if the extended release of a hydrophilic drug is required, since most of the suitable polymers for this are hydrophobic. Similarly, since hydrophilic polymers are used for fast-dissolving systems, it can be difficult to incorporate hydrophobic entities into these. Emulsion electrospinning was used to overcome the latter issue in the case of the lipophilic API celecoxib.[87] Emulsion droplets could be seen in the fibres produced and the drug was amorphously distributed in the fibres, boding well for improved dissolution properties (although these were not tested). The situation of a hydrophilic drug in a hydrophobic polymer has been studied by Ramakrishna's team.[88] Emulsion and blend fibres of PCL or poly(3-hydroxybutyric acid-co-3-hydroxyvaleric acid) (PHBV) loaded with metformin hydrochloride or metoprolol tartrate were generated,

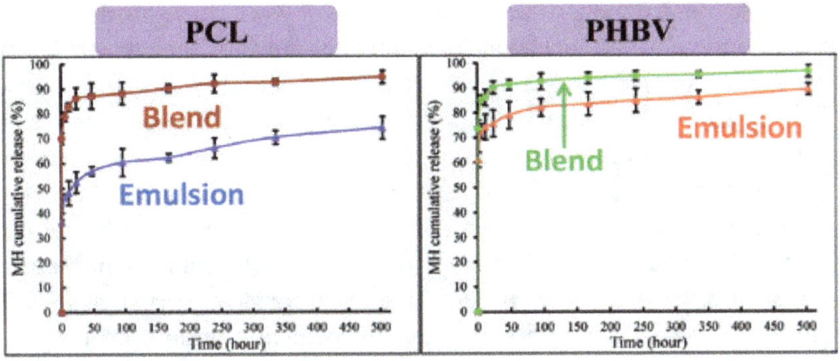

Figure 3.10 The release of metformin hydrochloride (MH) from blend and emulsion poly(ε-caprolactone) (PCL) and poly(3-hydroxybutyric acid-co-3-hydroxyvaleric acid) (PHBV) fibres. Reduced burst release and slower rates are seen with the emulsion system. (Reproduced with permission from Hu, J.; Prabhakaran, M. P.; Tian, L.; Ding, X.; Ramakrishna, S. 'Drug-loaded emulsion electrospun nanofibers: characterization, drug release and *in vitro* biocompatibility.' *RSC Adv.* 5 (2015): 100256–100267.[88] Copyright Royal Society of Chemistry 2015.)

and the initial burst and release rate were both reduced in the emulsion system (Figure 3.10).

It is not always the case that fibres made by emulsion electrospinning are superior to those from monoaxial solution spinning, however. A study by Zhao *et al.* fabricated PCL fibres loaded with L-ascorbic acid-2-phosphate magnesium using standard blend spinning (using a co-dissolving solution of drug and polymer), as well as with emulsion and coaxial electrospinning.[89] In this instance, the optimum fibres spun from solutions were found to have better mechanical properties and a reduced burst of release than the emulsion analogue.

3.11.2 Suspensions

Suspensions of small (typically nanoscale) particles can be converted into fibres by electrospinning. For example, $CaCO_3$ microparticles incorporating model drugs have been embedded in PLGA fibres by electrospinning.[90] The fibres appeared beaded owing to the presence of particles. However, it is possible to prepare relatively smooth cylindrical fibres with minimal beading, if the experimental conditions are appropriately optimised.[91]

Magnetic nanoparticles, such as those of Fe_3O_4, have attracted particular attention for inclusion into fibres, because of their potential in biosensing, imaging and cancer treatment (e.g. inducing magnetic hyperthermia to destroy cancer cells).[92] Wang *et al.* produced systems made of cellulose derivatives and containing Fe_3O_4 nanoparticles as well as either indomethacin or aspirin.[93] This resulted in magnetic fibres, but the inclusion of nanoparticles did not affect drug release. Other inorganic materials to have been electrospun include hydroxyapatite (useful for bone repair applications),[94] clays,[95] drug-loaded metal hydroxide nanoparticles[96] and silicas.[97] Jalvandi *et al.* have shown that by covalently binding levofloxacin to mesoporous silica nanoparticles and then spinning these into PCL fibres, drug release can be slowed and the initial burst reduced, compared to PCL/levofloxacin fibres with no nanoparticles present.[98]

Protein nanoparticles can also be prepared to help prevent degradation. This has been demonstrated by first encapsulating bone morphogenetic protein-2 (BMP-2) in BSA nanoparticles, and then electrospinning these into fibres based on poly(ε-caprolactone-co-poly(ethylene glycol)).[99] The rationale for this is that the BMP-2 is fragile, and could become degraded during electrospinning if processed in solution. Incorporating it into the BSA particles can protect it from degradation. This approach was found to give formulations able to repair defects in the skull of rats.

Finally, although most commonly researchers work with mixed solutions of a drug and polymer to generate fibres in the form of ASDs, it is also possible to electrospin suspensions of API particles.[100] This could be attractive for making extended-release systems, for instance.

3.12 Tissue-engineering applications

Electrospun fibres have attracted much attention for tissue-engineering applications, where they are explored as scaffolds to replace or heal biological tissue. The structure of the mat mimics the structural component of the extracellular matrix, a scaffold or network of nanofibrous proteins and gels of polysaccharides secreted by cells to give mechanical support to surrounding cells. This, coupled with the porosity of the mats (which means that nutrients and cellular waste can diffuse in and out, and it is possible for cells to infiltrate into the scaffold), can encourage cell growth. The fibres can be loaded with promoters of cell growth if required, and other functional ingredients (e.g. to prevent infection and modulate the inflammatory response toward regeneration rather than repair) may also be incorporated. Some examples of this are discussed above in the context of drug delivery.

For tissue engineering, the release from the fibres of a functional molecule may well be important, but the mechanical properties are also vital (they must mimic the relevant native tissue). Increasingly, researchers are seeking to make *bioresorbable scaffolds*, materials which degrade slowly over time in the body and are replaced by the body's own tissue. There are myriad applications of such systems, including for instance in the treatment of congenital heart defects. For such resorbable scaffolds to be effective, the degradation time of the polymer and the rate at which it is replaced by native tissue will need to be carefully considered and controlled. A detailed discussion of electrospun fibres in tissue engineering lies outside the scope of this volume, but there are a number of recent reviews which summarise elegantly the state of the art.[101]

3.13 Using fibres as sacrificial templates

As well as being used directly for drug delivery purposes, electrospun fibres can be used as sacrificial templates to generate higher-order materials. Electrospinning is regarded as a *top-down* fabrication technique, because the structure of the macroscale spinneret is propagated through into solid fibres (that is, a macroscopic object is used to prepare smaller ones). Another way to prepare nanoscale objects is *bottom-up*, in which smaller building blocks (often atoms and molecules) are brought together to form aggregates (e.g. in molecular self-assembly). This is a powerful approach, but unfortunately it is highly time-consuming, low-yield and more expensive than the top-down route. It is also very difficult to ensure that the building blocks assemble in the desired configuration. For example, self-assembled nanofibres often take the form of discontinuous fragments of fibrils of different lengths.

Liposomes (artificial vesicles bounded by a lipid bilayer) are one type of nanoscale system typically prepared bottom-up. Liposomes have numerous applications, including the delivery of therapeutic and diagnostic agents. They self-assemble in aqueous media owing to their amphiphilic nature; the formation of liposomes minimises contact between hydrophobic and hydrophilic groups, and thus is thermodynamically favourable. However, liposomes are unstable over time and have a tendency to aggregate. Controlling the size of the liposomes formed can also be challenging. Often, templates are used to direct the self-assembly processes and drive them towards the desired structure. Electrospun fibres can be used as such templates.

Yu *et al.* were the first to report this,[102] making PVP fibres containing phosphatidyl choline (PC), an amphiphilic molecule with a polar head

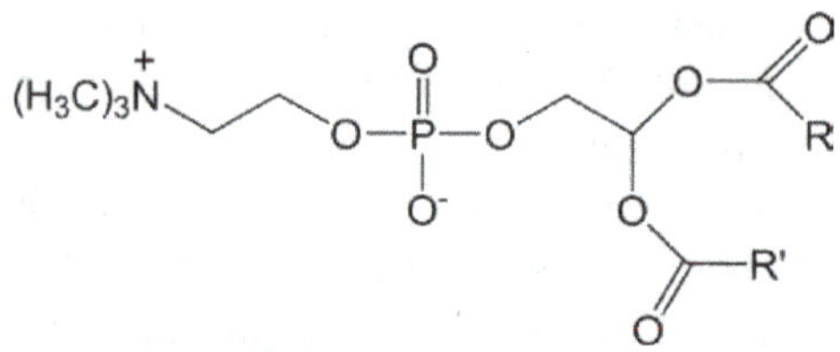

Figure 3.11 The chemical structure of phosphatidyl choline. R and R′ are long-chain fatty acid groups.

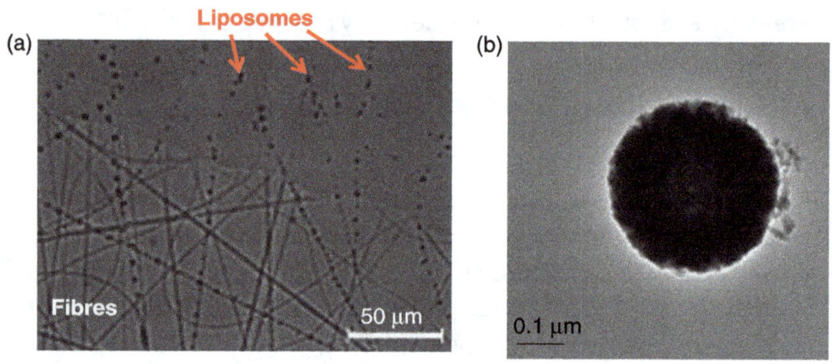

Figure 3.12 The self-assembly of phosphatidyl choline liposomes from poly(vinyl pyrrolidone)/phosphatidyl choline fibres, as reported by Yu *et al.*[102] (a) An optical microscopy image obtained during the self-assembly process, and (b) a transmission electron microscopy image of one of the resultant liposomes. (Reproduced with permission from Yu, D.-G.; Branford-White, C.; Williams, G. R.; Bligh, S. W. A.; White, K.; Zhu, L.-M.; Chatterton, N. P. 'Self-assembled liposomes from amphiphilic electrospun nanofibers.' *Soft Matter* 7 (2011): 8239–8247. Copyright Royal Society of Chemistry 2011.)

group and hydrophobic hydrocarbon tail (Figure 3.11). Amorphous solid dispersions of PC in PVP were obtained from electrospinning. When the fibres were added to water, the PC molecules were observed to self-assemble into liposomes (Figure 3.12), the size of which could be tuned by varying the fibre composition. The authors attributed this to the PVP matrix confining the PC molecules in close proximity when the fibres are

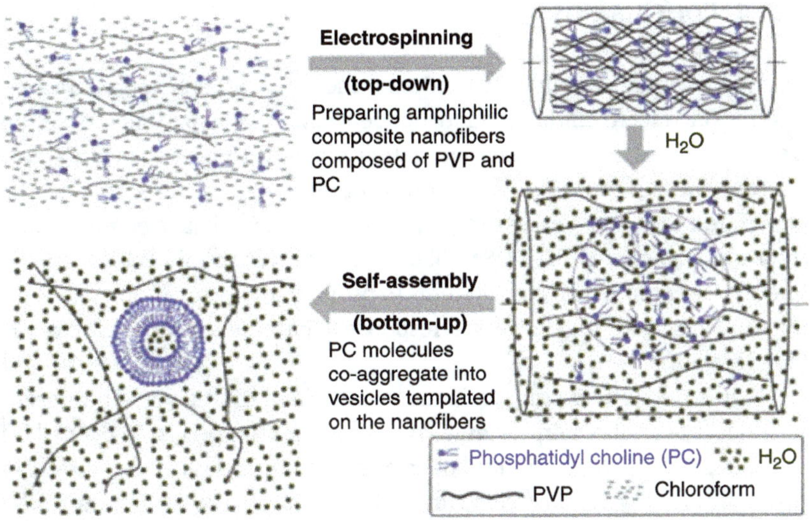

Figure 3.13 The proposed mechanism for liposome assembly from poly(vinyl pyrrolidone) (PVP)/phosphatidyl choline (PC) fibres. (Reproduced with permission from Yu, D.-G.; Branford-White, C.; Williams, G. R.; Bligh, S. W. A.; White, K.; Zhu, L.-M.; Chatterton, N. P. 'Self-assembled liposomes from amphiphilic electrospun nanofibers.' *Soft Matter* 7 (2011): 8239–8247. Copyright Royal Society of Chemistry 2011.)

added to water, driving them to aggregate into liposomes (Figure 3.13). This approach is potentially beneficial over other liposome production techniques, since it does not require any controlled heating, cooling or agitation steps. Furthermore, it can ameliorate some of the stability issues which are encountered during the storage of liposomes, because the fibres can act as proto-liposomes. These liposome precursors can be stored 'frozen' in the solid-state nanofibres, endowing them with high stability, but can easily be converted to liquid suspensions *in situ* upon demand.[102]

This work was developed further by Song and co-workers, who developed magnetic liposomes via a similar route.[103] Magnetic iron oxide nanoparticles were included in the fibres along with PVP and PC, and magnetic liposomes formed spontaneously when the fibres were added to water. The liposome size could be controlled by varying the iron oxide content of the fibres. The magnetic properties of the nanoparticles were unaffected by both the electrospinning and self-assembly processes, and thus these materials might find applications in targeted drug delivery.

3.14 Conclusions

In this chapter, we have considered the uses of fibres prepared by monoaxial electrospinning in drug delivery. The experimental set-up required was first explained, and details given as to how to begin a new electrospinning process. The various different types of fibres that can be generated were then discussed. Fibres made by monoaxial electrospinning find applications as FD-DDSs able to provide very rapid release in the mouth, as extended-release systems to prolong release over time, and can be used to target drug delivery in response to particular temperature or pH conditions.

It is possible to prepare fibre mats made of multilayers of different drug-carrying polymers to give more complex or precisely controlled drug delivery patterns, and suspensions and emulsions can be processed in addition to solutions; this can be beneficial in preventing an initial burst release of drug and protecting proteins from degradation. Finally, the potential to use the fibres as templates to self-assemble higher-order objects was considered.

Monoaxial spinning is the simplest electrospinning technique and thus has received a great deal of attention in the literature, with many promising applications. However, there are some drawbacks – in particular the burst of drug release which is often seen at the beginning of experiments – and therefore in some instances more complex approaches are required. We will discuss these in Chapters 4 and 5.

3.15 References

1. Kenawy, E.-R.; Bowlin, G. L.; Mansfield, K.; Layman, J.; Simpson, D. G.; Sanders, E. H.; Wnek, G. E. 'Release of tetracycline hydrochloride from electrospun poly(ethylene-co-vinylacetate), poly(lactic acid), and a blend.' *J. Control. Release* 81 (2002): 57–64.
2. (a) Chou, S.-F.; Carson, D.; Woodrow, K. A. 'Current strategies for sustaining drug release from electrospun nanofibers.' *J. Control. Release* 220 (2015): 584–591; (b) Krogstad, E. A.; Woodrow, K. A. 'Manufacturing scale-up of electrospun poly(vinyl alcohol) fibers containing tenofovir for vaginal drug delivery.' *Int. J. Pharm.* 475 (2014): 282–291; (c) Ball, C.; Woodrow, K. A. 'Electrospun solid dispersions of maraviroc for rapid intravaginal preexposure prophylaxis of HIV.' *Antimicrob. Agents Chemother.* 58 (2014): 4855–4865; (d) Blakney, A. K.; Krogstad, E. A.; Jiang, Y. H.; Woodrow, K. A. 'Delivery of multipurpose prevention drug combinations

from electrospun nanofibers using composite microarchitectures.' *Int. J. Nanomedicine* 9 (2014): 2967–2978.

3. (a) Ball, C.; Krogstad, E.; Chaowanachan, T.; Woodrow, K. A. 'Drug-eluting fibers for HIV-1 inhibition and contraception.' *PLoS ONE* 7 (2012): e49792; (b) Blakney, A. K.; Ball, C.; Krogstad, E. A.; Woodrow, K. A. 'Electrospun fibers for vaginal anti-HIV drug delivery.' *Antiviral Res.* 100 (2013): S9–S16.
4. (a) Pelipenko, J.; Kocbek, P.; Kristl, J. 'Critical attributes of nanofibers: Preparation, drug loading, and tissue regeneration.' *Int. J. Pharm.* 484 (2015): 57–74; (b) Zupančič, Š.; Sinha-Ray, S.; Sinha-Ray, S.; Kristl, J.; Yarin, A. L. 'Long-term sustained ciprofloxacin release from PMMA and hydrophilic polymer blended nanofibers.' *Mol. Pharm.* 13 (2016): 295–305; (c) Falde, E. J.; Freedman, J. D.; Herrera, V. L. M.; Yohe, S. T.; Colson, Y. L.; Grinstaff, M. W. 'Layered superhydrophobic meshes for controlled drug release.' *J. Control. Release* 214 (2015): 23–29.
5. Williams, G. R.; Chatterton, N. P.; Nazir, T.; Yu, D.-G.; Zhu, L.-M.; Branford-White, C. J. 'Electrospun nanofibers in drug delivery: Recent developments and perspectives.' *Therap. Deliv.* 3 (2012): 515–533.
6. Krogstad, E. A.; Rathbone, M. J.; Woodrow, K. A., 'Vaginal drug delivery.' In *Focal Controlled Drug Delivery*, edited by Domb, A. J.; Khan, W., 607–651. Boston: Springer US, 2014.
7. Chakraborty, S.; Liao, I. C.; Adler, A.; Leong, K. W. 'Electrohydrodynamics: A facile technique to fabricate drug delivery systems.' *Adv. Drug Deliv. Rev.* 61 (2009): 1043–1054.
8. Katsogiannis, K. A. G.; Vladisavljević, G. T.; Georgiadou, S. 'Porous electrospun polycaprolactone (PCL) fibres by phase separation.' *Eur. Polym. J.* 69 (2015): 284–295.
9. Xiang, Q.; Ma, Y.-M.; Yu, D.-G.; Jin, M.; Williams, G. R. 'Electrospinning using a Teflon-coated spinneret.' *Appl. Surf. Sci.* 284 (2013): 889–893.
10. Wang, X.; Li, X.-Y.; Li, Y.; Zou, H.; Yu, D. G.; Cai, J.-S. 'Electrospun acetaminophen-loaded cellulose acetate nanofibers fabricated using an epoxy-coated spinneret.' *e-Polymers* 15 (2015): 311–315.
11. Chuangchote, S.; Sagawa, T.; Yoshikawa, S. 'Electrospinning of poly(vinyl pyrrolidone): Effects of solvents on electrospinnability for the fabrication of poly(p-phenylene vinylene) and TiO_2 nanofibers.' *J. Appl. Polym. Sci.* 114 (2009): 2777–2791.
12. Leach, M. K.; Z.Q., F.; Tuck, S. J.; Corey, J. M. 'Electrospinning fundamentals: Optimizing solution and apparatus parameters.' *J. Vis. Exp.* 47 (2011): e2494.
13. Sill, T. J.; von Recum, H. A. 'Electrospinning: Applications in drug delivery and tissue engineering.' *Biomaterials* 29 (2008): 1989–2006.
14. Acatay, K.; Simsek, E.; Ow-Yang, C.; Menceloglu, Y. Z. 'Tunable, superhydrophobically stable polymeric surfaces by electrospinning.' *Angew. Chem.* 116 (2004): 5322–5325.
15. (a) Deitzel, J. M.; Kleinmeyer, J.; Harris, D.; Beck Tan, N. C. 'The effect of processing variables on the morphology of electrospun nanofibers and textiles.'

Polymer 42 (2001): 261–272; (b) Garg, K.; Bowlin, G. L. 'Electrospinning jets and nanofibrous structures.' *Biomicrofluidics* 5 (2011): 013403.

16. Brown, T. D.; Dalton, P. D.; Hutmacher, D. W. 'Direct writing by way of melt electrospinning.' *Adv. Mater.* 23 (2011): 5651–5657.
17. Liang, D.; Hsiao, B. S.; Chu, B. 'Functional electrospun nanofibrous scaffolds for biomedical applications.' *Adv. Drug Deliv. Rev.* 59 (2007): 1392–1412.
18. Lopez, F. L.; Shearman, G. C.; Gaisford, S.; Williams, G. R. 'Amorphous formulations of indomethacin and griseofulvin prepared by electrospinning.' *Mol. Pharm.* 11 (2014): 4327–4338.
19. (a) Chaudhary, H.; Gauri, S.; Rathee, P.; Kumar, V. 'Development and optimization of fast dissolving oro-dispersible films of granisetron HCl using Box–Behnken statistical design.' *Bull. Fac. Pharm. Cairo Univ.* 51 (2013): 193–201; (b) Hoffmann, E. M.; Breitenbach, A.; Breitkreutz, J. 'Advances in orodispersible films for drug delivery.' *Expert Op. Drug Del.* 8 (2011): 299–316; (c) Illangakoon, U. E.; Gill, H.; Shearman, G. C.; Parhizkar, M.; Mahalingam, S.; Chatterton, N. P.; Williams, G. R. 'Fast dissolving paracetamol/caffeine nanofibers prepared by electrospinning.' *Int. J. Pharm.* 477 (2014): 369–379.
20. Seager, H. 'Drug-delivery products and the Zydis fast-dissolving dosage form.' *J. Pharm. Pharmacol.* 50 (1998): 375–382.
21. Yu, D. G.; Shen, X. X.; Branford-White, C.; White, K.; Zhu, L. M.; Bligh, S. W. 'Oral fast-dissolving drug delivery membranes prepared from electrospun polyvinylpyrrolidone ultrafine fibers.' *Nanotechnology* 20 (2009): 055104.
22. Adeli, E. 'Irbesartan-loaded electrospun nanofibers-based PVP K90 for the drug dissolution improvement: Fabrication, *in vitro* performance assessment, and *in vivo* evaluation.' *J. Appl. Polym. Sci.* 132 (2015): 42212.
23. Yu, D.-G.; Branford-White, C.; Shen, X.-X.; Zhang, X.-F.; Zhu, L.-M. 'Solid dispersions of ketoprofen in drug-loaded electrospun nanofibers.' *J. Dispersion Sci. Technol.* 31 (2010): 902–908.
24. Illangakoon, U. E.; Nazir, T.; Williams, G. R.; Chatterton, N. P. 'Mebeverine-loaded electrospun nanofibers: Physicochemical characterization and dissolution studies.' *J. Pharm. Sci.* 103 (2014): 283–292.
25. Li, X.; Lin, L.; Zhu, Y.; Liu, W.; Yu, T.; Ge, M. 'Preparation of ultrafine fast-dissolving cholecalciferol-loaded poly(vinyl pyrrolidone) fiber mats via electrospinning.' *Polym. Composite.* 34 (2013): 282–287.
26. Chen, J.; Wang, X.; Zhang, W.; Yu, S.; Fan, J.; Cheng, B.; Yang, X.; Pan, W. 'A novel application of electrospinning technique in sublingual membrane: Characterization, permeation and *in vivo* study.' *Drug. Dev. Ind. Pharm.* 42 (2016): 1365–1374.
27. Li, X.-Y.; Wang, X.; Yu, D.-G.; Ye, S.; Kuang, Q.-K.; Yi, Q.-W.; Yao, X.-Z. 'Electrospun borneol–PVP nanocomposites.' *J. Nanomater.* 2012 (2012): 731382.
28. Wang, C.; Ma, C.; Wu, Z.; Liang, H.; Yan, P.; Song, J.; Ma, N.; Zhao, Q. 'Enhanced bioavailability and anticancer effect of curcumin-loaded electrospun nanofiber: *In vitro* and *in vivo* study.' *Nanoscale Res. Lett.* 10 (2015): 439.

29. Li, X.; Kanjwal, M. A.; Lin, L.; Chronakis, I. S. 'Electrospun polyvinyl-alcohol nanofibers as oral fast-dissolving delivery system of caffeine and riboflavin.' *Colloids Surf. B* 103 (2013): 182–188.
30. Krstic, M.; Radojevic, M.; Stojanovic, D.; Radojevic, V.; Uskokovic, P.; Ibric, S. 'Formulation and characterization of nanofibers and films with carvedilol prepared by electrospinning and solution casting method.' *Eur. J. Pharm. Sci.* 101 (2017): 160–166.
31. Taepaiboon, P.; Rungsardthong, U.; Supaphol, P. 'Drug-loaded electrospun mats of poly(vinyl alcohol) fibres and their release characteristics of four model drugs.' *Nanotechnol.* 17 (2006): 2317–2329.
32. Rasekh, M.; Karavasili, C.; Soong, Y. L.; Bouropoulos, N.; Morris, M.; Armitage, D.; Li, X.; Fatouros, D. G.; Ahmad, Z. 'Electrospun PVP–indomethacin constituents for transdermal dressings and drug delivery devices.' *Int. J. Pharm.* 473 (2014): 95–104.
33. Baskakova, A.; Awwad, S.; Jimenez, J. Q.; Gill, H.; Novikov, O.; Khaw, P. T.; Brocchini, S.; Zhilyakova, E.; Williams, G. R. 'Electrospun formulations of acyclovir, ciprofloxacin and cyanocobalamin for ocular drug delivery.' *Int. J. Pharm.* 502 (2016): 208–218.
34. Samprasit, W.; Akkaramongkolporn, P.; Ngawhirunpat, T.; Rojanarata, T.; Kaomongkolgit, R.; Opanasopit, P. 'Fast releasing oral electrospun PVP/CD nanofiber mats of taste-masked meloxicam.' *Int. J. Pharm.* 487 (2015): 213–222.
35. Vrbata, P.; Berka, P.; Stranska, D.; Dolezal, P.; Musilova, M.; Cizinska, L. 'Electrospun drug loaded membranes for sublingual administration of sumatriptan and naproxen.' *Int. J. Pharm.* 457 (2013): 168–176.
36. Yu, D.-G.; Yang, J.-M.; Branford-White, C.; Lu, P.; Zhang, L.; Zhu, L.-M. 'Third generation solid dispersions of ferulic acid in electrospun composite nanofibers.' *Int. J. Pharm.* 400 (2010): 158–164.
37. Brettmann, B. K.; Myerson, A. S.; Trout, B. L. 'Solid-state nuclear magnetic resonance study of the physical stability of electrospun drug and polymer solid solutions.' *J. Pharm. Sci.* 101 (2012): 2185–2193.
38. Demuth, B.; Farkas, A.; Pataki, H.; Balogh, A.; Szabo, B.; Borbas, E.; Soti, P. L.; Vigh, T.; Kiserdei, E.; Farkas, B.; Mensch, J.; Verreck, G.; Van Assche, I.; Marosi, G.; Nagy, Z. K. 'Detailed stability investigation of amorphous solid dispersions prepared by single-needle and high speed electrospinning.' *Int. J. Pharm.* 498 (2016): 234–244.
39. Tiwari, S. B.; Rajabi-Siahboomi, A. R., 'Extended-release oral drug delivery technologies: Monolithic matrix systems.' In *Drug Delivery Systems*, edited by Jain, K. K., 217–243. Totowa: Humana Press, 2008.
40. Bhardwaj, N.; Kundu, S. C. 'Electrospinning: A fascinating fiber fabrication technique.' *Biotechnol. Adv.* 28 (2010): 325–347.
41. (a) Piskin, E.; Bölgen, N.; Egri, S.; Isoglu, I. A. 'Electrospun matrices made of poly(α-hydroxy acids) for medical use.' *Nanomedicine* 2 (2007): 441–457; (b) Schiffman, J. D.; Schauer, C. L. 'A review: Electrospinning of biopolymer nanofibers and their applications.' *Polym. Rev.* 48 (2008): 317–352.

42. Xie, J.; Wang, C. H. 'Electrospun micro- and nanofibers for sustained delivery of paclitaxel to treat C6 glioma *in vitro*.' *Pharm. Res.* 23 (2006): 1817–1826.
43. Xie, J.; Tan, R. S.; Wang, C. H. 'Biodegradable microparticles and fiber fabrics for sustained delivery of cisplatin to treat C6 glioma *in vitro*.' *J. Biomed. Mater. Res. A* 85 (2008): 897–908.
44. Park, Y.; Kang, E.; Kwon, O. J.; Hwang, T.; Park, H.; Lee, J. M.; Kim, J. H.; Yun, C. O. 'Ionically crosslinked Ad/chitosan nanocomplexes processed by electrospinning for targeted cancer gene therapy.' *J. Control. Release* 148 (2010): 75–82.
45. Puppi, D.; Piras, A. M.; Detta, N.; Dinucci, D.; Chiellini, F. 'Poly(lactic-co-glycolic acid) electrospun fibrous meshes for the controlled release of retinoic acid.' *Acta Biomater.* 6 (2010): 1258–1268.
46. Luong-Van, E.; Grondahl, L.; Chua, K. N.; Leong, K. W.; Nurcombe, V.; Cool, S. M. 'Controlled release of heparin from poly(epsilon-caprolactone) electrospun fibers.' *Biomaterials* 27 (2006): 2042–2050.
47. Hall Barrientos, I. J.; Paladino, E.; Brozio, S.; Passarelli, M. K.; Moug, S.; Black, R. A.; Wilson, C. G.; Lamprou, D. A. 'Fabrication and characterisation of drug-loaded electrospun polymeric nanofibers for controlled release in hernia repair.' *Int. J. Pharm.* 517 (2017): 329–337.
48. Zhang, Z.; Tang, J.; Wang, H.; Xia, Q.; Xu, S.; Han, C. C. 'Controlled antibiotics release system through simple blended electrospun fibers for sustained antibacterial effects.' *ACS Appl. Mater. Interfaces* 7 (2015): 26400–26404.
49. Jiang, J.; Chen, G.; Shuler, F. D.; Wang, C. H.; Xie, J. 'Local sustained delivery of 25-hydroxyvitamin D3 for production of antimicrobial peptides.' *Pharm. Res.* 32 (2015): 2851–2862.
50. He, T.; Wang, J.; Huang, P.; Zeng, B.; Li, H.; Cao, Q.; Zhang, S.; Luo, Z.; Deng, D. Y.; Zhang, H.; Zhou, W. 'Electrospinning polyvinylidene fluoride fibrous membranes containing anti-bacterial drugs used as wound dressing.' *Colloids Surf. B* 130 (2015): 278–286.
51. Zamani, M.; Morshed, M.; Varshosaz, J.; Jannesari, M. 'Controlled release of metronidazole benzoate from poly epsilon-caprolactone electrospun nanofibers for periodontal diseases.' *Eur. J. Pharm. Biopharm.* 75 (2010): 179–185.
52. Yu, D.-G.; Branford-White, C.; Li, L.; Wu, X.-M.; Zhu, L.-M. 'The compatibility of acyclovir with polyacrylonitrile in the electrospun drug-loaded nanofibers.' *J. Appl. Polym. Sci.* (2010): 1509–1515.
53. Lu, H.; Wang, Q.; Li, G.; Qiu, Y.; Wei, Q. 'Electrospun water-stable zein/ethyl cellulose composite nanofiber and its drug release properties.' *Mater. Sci. Eng. C* 74 (2017): 86–93.
54. Jalvandi, J.; White, M.; Gao, Y.; Truong, Y. B.; Padhye, R.; Kyratzis, I. L. 'Polyvinyl alcohol composite nanofibres containing conjugated levofloxacin–chitosan for controlled drug release.' *Mater. Sci. Eng. C* 73 (2017): 440–446.

55. Natu, M. V.; de Sousa, H. C.; Gil, M. H. 'Effects of drug solubility, state and loading on controlled release in bicomponent electrospun fibers.' *Int. J. Pharm.* 397 (2010): 50–58.
56. Verreck, G.; Chun, I.; Peeters, J.; Rosenblatt, J.; Brewster, M. E. 'Preparation and characterization of nanofibers containing amorphous drug dispersions generated by electrostatic spinning.' *Pharm. Res.* 20 (2003): 810–817.
57. Xie, Z.; Buschle-Diller, G. 'Electrospun poly(D,L-lactide) fibers for drug delivery: The influence of cosolvent and the mechanism of drug release.' *J. Appl. Polym. Sci.* 115 (2010): 1–8.
58. Zamani, M.; Prabhakaran, M. P.; Ramakrishna, S. 'Advances in drug delivery via electrospun and electrosprayed nanomaterials.' *Int. J. Nanomedicine* 8 (2013): 2997–3017.
59. Wang, M.; Wang, L.; Huang, Y. 'Electrospun hydroxypropyl methyl cellulose phthalate (HPMCP)/erythromycin fibers for targeted release in intestine.' *J. Appl. Polym. Sci.* 106 (2007): 2177–2184.
60. Shen, X.; Yu, D.; Zhu, L.; Branford-White, C.; White, K.; Chatterton, N. P. 'Electrospun diclofenac sodium loaded Eudragit L100–55 nanofibers for colon-targeted drug delivery.' *Int. J. Pharm.* 408 (2011): 200–207.
61. Akhgari, A.; Heshmati, Z.; Afrasiabi Garekani, H.; Sadeghi, F.; Sabbagh, A.; Sharif Makhmalzadeh, B.; Nokhodchi, A. 'Indomethacin electrospun nanofibers for colonic drug delivery: *In vitro* dissolution studies.' *Colloids Surf. B* 152 (2017): 29–35.
62. Karthikeyan, K.; Guhathakarta, S.; Rajaram, R.; Korrapati, P. S. 'Electrospun zein/eudragit nanofibers based dual drug delivery system for the simultaneous delivery of aceclofenac and pantoprazole.' *Int. J. Pharm.* 438 (2012): 117–122.
63. Zhao, J.; Jiang, S.; Zheng, R.; Zhao, X.; Chen, X.; Fan, C.; Cui, W. 'Smart electrospun fibrous scaffolds inhibit tumor cells and promote normal cell proliferation.' *RSC Adv.* 4 (2014): 51696–51702.
64. Zhao, J. W.; Cui, W. G. 'Fabrication of acid-responsive electrospun fibers via doping sodium bicarbonate for quick releasing drug.' *Nanosci. Nanotechnol. Lett.* 6 (2014): 339–345.
65. Salehi, R.; Irani, M.; Eskandani, M.; Nowruzi, K.; Davaran, S.; Haririan, I. 'Interaction, controlled release, and antitumor activity of doxorubicin hydrochloride from pH-sensitive p(NIPAAm-MAA-VP) nanofibrous scaffolds prepared by green electrospinning.' *Int. J. Polym. Mater.* 63 (2014): 609–619.
66. Kaassis, A. Y. A.; Young, N.; Sano, N.; Merchant, H. A.; Yu, D.-G.; Chatterton, N. P.; Williams, G. R. 'Pulsatile drug release from electrospun poly(ethylene oxide)–sodium alginate blend nanofibres.' *J. Mater. Chem. B* 2 (2014): 1400–1407.
67. Alhusein, N.; Blagbrough, I. S.; De Bank, P. A. 'Electrospun matrices for localised controlled drug delivery: Release of tetracycline hydrochloride from layers of polycaprolactone and poly(ethylene-co-vinyl acetate).' *Drug Deliv. Trans. Res.* 2 (2012): 477–488.

68. Alhusein, N.; De Bank, P. A.; Blagbrough, I. S.; Bolhuis, A. 'Killing bacteria within biofilms by sustained release of tetracycline from triple-layered electrospun micro/nanofibre matrices of polycaprolactone and poly(ethylene-co-vinyl acetate).' *Drug Del. Trans. Res.* 3 (2013): 531–541.
69. Alhusein, N.; Blagbrough, I. S.; De Bank, P. A. 'Zein/polycaprolactone electrospun matrices for localised controlled delivery of tetracycline.' *Drug Del. Trans. Res.* 3 (2013): 542–550.
70. Alhusein, N.; Blagbrough, I. S.; Beeton, M. L.; Bolhuis, A.; De Bank, P. A. 'Electrospun zein/PCL fibrous matrices release tetracycline in a controlled manner, killing *Staphylococcus aureus* both in biofilms and *ex vivo* on pig skin, and are compatible with human skin cells.' *Pharm. Res.* 33 (2016): 237–246.
71. Huang, L. Y.; Branford-White, C.; Shen, X. X.; Yu, D. G.; Zhu, L. M. 'Time-engineeringed biphasic drug release by electrospun nanofiber meshes.' *Int. J. Pharm.* 436 (2012): 88–96.
72. Rockwood, D. N.; Chase, D. B.; Akins, R. E.; Rabolt, J. F. 'Characterization of electrospun poly(*N*-isopropyl acrylamide) fibers.' *Polymer* 49 (2008): 4025–4032.
73. (a) Wang, N.; Zhao, Y.; Jiang, L. 'Low-cost, thermoresponsive wettability of surfaces: Poly(*N*-isopropylacrylamide)/polystyrene composite films prepared by electrospinning.' *Macromol. Rapid Commun.* 29 (2008): 485–489; (b) Gu, S.-Y.; Wang, Z.-M.; Li, J.-B.; Ren, J. 'Switchable wettability of thermo-responsive biocompatible nanofibrous films created by electrospinning.' *Macromol. Mater. Eng.* 295 (2010): 32–36.
74. Lin, X.; Tang, D.; Cui, W.; Cheng, Y. 'Controllable drug release of electrospun thermoresponsive poly(*N*-isopropylacrylamide)/poly(2-acrylamido-2-methyl-propanesulfonic acid) nanofibers.' *J. Biomed. Mater. Res. A* 100 (2012): 1839–1845.
75. Song, F.; Wang, X. L.; Wang, Y. Z. 'Poly (*N*-isopropylacrylamide)/poly (ethylene oxide) blend nanofibrous scaffolds: Thermo-responsive carrier for controlled drug release.' *Colloids Surf. B* 88 (2011): 749–754.
76. Hu, J.; Li, H.-Y.; Williams, G. R.; Yang, H.-H.; Tao, L.; Zhu, L.-M. 'Electrospun poly(*N*-isopropylacrylamide)/ethyl cellulose nanofibers as thermoresponsive drug delivery systems.' *J. Pharm. Sci.* 105 (2016).
77. Li, H.; Williams, G. R.; Wu, J.; Wang, H.; Sun, X.; Zhu, L. M. 'Poly(N-isopropylacrylamide)/poly(L-lactic acid-co-caprolactone) fibers loaded with ciprofloxacin as wound dressing materials.' *Mater. Sci. Eng. C* 79 (2017): 245–254.
78. Li, H.; Williams, G. R.; Wu, J.; Lv, Y.; Sun, X.; Wu, H.; Zhu, L. M. 'Thermosensitive nanofibers loaded with ciprofloxacin as antibacterial wound dressing materials.' *Int. J. Pharm.* 517 (2017): 135–147.
79. Xu, X.; Chen, X.; Ma, P.; Wang, X.; Jing, X. 'The release behavior of doxorubicin hydrochloride from medicated fibers prepared by emulsion-electrospinning.' *Eur. J. Pharm. Biopharm.* 70 (2008): 165–170.

80. Wang, C.; Wang, M. 'Formation of core–shell structures in emulsion electrospun fibres: A comparative study.' *Aust. J. Chem.* 67 (2014): 1403–1413.
81. Hu, J.; Wei, J.; Liu, W.; Chen, Y. 'Preparation and characterization of electrospun PLGA/gelatin nanofibers as a drug delivery system by emulsion electrospinning.' *J. Biomater. Sci. Polym. Ed.* 24 (2013): 972–985.
82. Sy, J. C.; Klemm, A. S.; Shastri, V. P. 'Emulsion as a means of controlling electrospinning of polymers.' *Adv. Mater.* 21 (2009): 1814–1819.
83. (a) Yang, Y.; Li, X.; He, S.; Cheng, L.; Chen, F.; Zhou, S.; Weng, J. 'Biodegradable ultrafine fibers with core–sheath structures for protein delivery and its optimization.' *Polym. Adv. Technol.* 22 (2011): 1842–1850; (b) Briggs, T.; Arinzeh, T. L. 'Examining the formulation of emulsion electrospinning for improving the release of bioactive proteins from electrospun fibers.' *J. Biomed. Mater. Res. A* 102 (2014): 674–684.
84. Yang, Y.; Li, X.; Cui, W.; Zhou, S.; Tan, R.; Wang, C. 'Structural stability and release profiles of proteins from core–shell poly (DL-lactide) ultrafine fibers prepared by emulsion electrospinning.' *J. Biomed. Mater. Res. A* 86 (2008): 374–385.
85. Tian, L.; Prabhakaran, M. P.; Ding, X.; Kai, D.; Ramakrishna, S. 'Emulsion electrospun vascular endothelial growth factor encapsulated poly(L-lactic acid-co-ε-caprolactone) nanofibers for sustained release in cardiac tissue engineering.' *J. Mater. Sci.* 47 (2011): 3272–3281.
86. (a) Tian, L.; Prabhakaran, M. P.; Ding, X.; Ramakrishna, S. 'Biocompatibility evaluation of emulsion electrospun nanofibers using osteoblasts for bone tissue engineering.' *J. Biomater. Sci. Polym. Ed.* 24 (2013): 1952–1968; (b) Spano, F.; Quarta, A.; Martelli, C.; Ottobrini, L.; Rossi, R. M.; Gigli, G.; Blasi, L. 'Fibrous scaffolds fabricated by emulsion electrospinning: From hosting capacity to *in vivo* biocompatibility.' *Nanoscale* 8 (2016): 9293–9303.
87. Gordon, V.; Marom, G.; Magdassi, S. 'Formation of hydrophilic nanofibers from nanoemulsions through electrospinning.' *Int. J. Pharm.* 478 (2015): 172–179.
88. Hu, J.; Prabhakaran, M. P.; Tian, L.; Ding, X.; Ramakrishna, S. 'Drug-loaded emulsion electrospun nanofibers: Characterization, drug release and *in vitro* biocompatibility.' *RSC Adv.* 5 (2015): 100256–100267.
89. Zhao, X.; Lui, Y.; Toh, P.; Loo, S. 'Sustained release of hydrophilic L-ascorbic acid 2-phosphate magnesium from electrospun polycaprolactone scaffold – a study across blend, coaxial, and emulsion electrospinning techniques.' *Materials* 7 (2014): 7398–7408.
90. Ma, J.; Meng, J.; Simonet, M.; Stingelin, N.; Peijs, T.; Sukhorukov, G. B. 'Biodegradable fibre scaffolds incorporating water-soluble drugs and proteins.' *J. Mater. Sci. Mater. Med.* 26 (2015): 205.
91. Li, K.; Sun, H.; Sui, H.; Zhang, Y.; Liang, H.; Wu, X.; Zhao, Q. 'Composite mesoporous silica nanoparticle/chitosan nanofibers for bone tissue engineering.' *RSC Adv.* 5 (2015): 17541–17549.

92. (a) Burke, L.; Mortimer, C. J.; Curtis, D. J.; Lewis, A. R.; Williams, R.; Hawkins, K.; Maffeis, T. G.; Wright, C. J. 'In-situ synthesis of magnetic iron-oxide nanoparticle–nanofibre composites using electrospinning.' *Mater. Sci. Eng. C* 70 (2017): 512–519; (b) Zhang, H.; Xia, J.; Pang, X.; Zhao, M.; Wang, B.; Yang, L.; Wan, H.; Wu, J.; Fu, S. 'Magnetic nanoparticle-loaded electrospun polymeric nanofibers for tissue engineering.' *Mater. Sci. Eng. C* 73 (2017): 537–543.
93. Wang, L.; Wang, M.; Topham, P. D.; Huang, Y. 'Fabrication of magnetic drug-loaded polymeric composite nanofibres and their drug release characteristics.' *RSC Adv.* 2 (2012): 2433.
94. Kim, H. W.; Lee, H. H.; Knowles, J. C. 'Electrospinning biomedical nanocomposite fibers of hydroxyapatite/poly(lactic acid) for bone regeneration.' *J. Biomed. Mater. Res. A* 79 (2006): 643–649.
95. Lee, I. W.; Li, J.; Chen, X.; Park, H. J. 'Electrospun poly(vinyl alcohol) composite nanofibers with halloysite nanotubes for the sustained release of sodium-pantothenate.' *J. Appl. Polym. Sci.* 133 (2016): 42900.
96. Valarezo, E.; Tammaro, L.; González, S.; Malagón, O.; Vittoria, V. 'Fabrication and sustained release properties of poly(ε-caprolactone) electrospun fibers loaded with layered double hydroxide nanoparticles intercalated with amoxicillin.' *Appl. Clay Sci.* 72 (2013): 104–109.
97. Fazli, Y.; Shariatinia, Z. 'Controlled release of cefazolin sodium antibiotic drug from electrospun chitosan–polyethylene oxide nanofibrous mats.' *Mater. Sci. Eng. C* 71 (2017): 641–652.
98. Jalvandi, J.; White, M.; Gao, Y.; Truong, Y. B.; Padhye, R.; Kyratzis, I. L. 'Slow release of levofloxacin conjugated on silica nanoparticles from poly (εcaprolactone) nanofibers.' *Int. J. Polym. Mater.* 66 (2017): 507–513.
99. Li, L.; Zhou, G.; Wang, Y.; Yang, G.; Ding, S.; Zhou, S. 'Controlled dual delivery of BMP-2 and dexamethasone by nanoparticle-embedded electrospun nanofibers for the efficient repair of critical-sized rat calvarial defect.' *Biomaterials* 37 (2015): 218–229.
100. Brettmann, B. K.; Cheng, K.; Myerson, A. S.; Trout, B. L. 'Electrospun formulations containing crystalline active pharmaceutical ingredients.' *Pharm. Res.* 30 (2013): 238–246.
101. (a) Haidar, M. K.; Eroglu, H. 'Nanofibers: New insights for drug delivery and tissue engineering.' *Curr. Top. Med. Chem.* 17 (2016): 1564–1579; (b) Kitsara, M.; Agbulut, O.; Kontziampasis, D.; Chen, Y.; Menasche, P. 'Fibers for hearts: A critical review on electrospinning for cardiac tissue engineering.' *Acta Biomater.* 48 (2017): 20–40; (c) Asghari, F.; Samiei, M.; Adibkia, K.; Akbarzadeh, A.; Davaran, S. 'Biodegradable and biocompatible polymers for tissue engineering application: A review.' *Artif. Cells Nanomed. Biotechnol.* 45 (2017): 185–192; (d) Rezvani, Z.; Venugopal, J. R.; Urbanska, A. M.; Mills, D. K.; Ramakrishna, S.; Mozafari, M. 'A bird's eye view on the use of electrospun nanofibrous scaffolds for bone tissue engineering: Current state-of-the-art, emerging directions and future trends.'

Nanomedicine 12 (2016): 2181–2200; (e) O'Connor, R. A.; McGuinness, G. B. 'Electrospun nanofibre bundles and yarns for tissue engineering applications: A review.' *Proc. Inst. Mech. Eng. H* 230 (2016): 987–998; (f) Kong, B.; Mi, S. 'Electrospun scaffolds for corneal tissue engineering: A review.' *Materials* 9 (2016): 614; (g) Khorshidi, S.; Solouk, A.; Mirzadeh, H.; Mazinani, S.; Lagaron, J. M.; Sharifi, S.; Ramakrishna, S. 'A review of key challenges of electrospun scaffolds for tissue-engineering applications.' *J. Tissue Eng. Regen. Med.* 10 (2016): 715–738.

102. Yu, D.-G.; Branford-White, C.; Williams, G. R.; Bligh, S. W. A.; White, K.; Zhu, L.-M.; Chatterton, N. P. 'Self-assembled liposomes from amphiphilic electrospun nanofibers.' *Soft Matter* 7 (2011): 8239–8247.
103. Song, H.-H.; Gong, X.; Williams, G. R.; Quan, J.; Nie, H.-L.; Zhu, L.-M.; Nan, E.-L.; Shao, M. 'Self-assembled magnetic liposomes from electrospun fibers.' *Mater. Res. Bull.* 53 (2014): 280–289.

4

Integration Coaxial and Multi-axial Electrospinning

4.1 Introduction

As discussed in Chapter 2 (section 2.6.3), coaxial electrospinning (also known as co-electrospinning) involves the use of a two-needle spinneret, with one needle nested inside another in a concentric fashion. The rapid stretching and solvent evaporation in electrospinning mean that the structure of the spinneret is propagated into the fibre products: thus, where the single-liquid, monoaxial, electrospinning process gives monolithic fibres, the arrangement of needles in coaxial spinning most commonly produces core/shell materials. This is depicted in Figure 4.1.

The first report of coaxial electrospinning in the literature appeared in 2003.[1] In this work Sun *et al.* described the spinning of systems where both the core and shell comprised poly(ethylene oxide) (PEO), in addition to materials comprising PEO (shell)/poly(dodecylthiophene) (core), PEO/polysulfone and poly(L-lactic acid) (PLLA)/palladium acetate.[1] It was noted in this work that it is possible to use solutions which are non-electrospinnable for the core so long as the shell solution is amenable to processing by electrospinning, thereby significantly broadening the range of materials which can be handled. It was subsequently found that non-electrospinnable solutions can also be used as shell liquid when paired with an electrospinnable core solution, as elaborated in section 4.9. Since the work by Sun *et al.*, there has been an explosion of interest in using coaxial electrospinning to prepare drug delivery systems.

Coaxial systems have a number of potential benefits over the monolithic fibres produced in single-liquid spinning. These include preventing the initial burst of release commonly seen with monolithic fibres, or

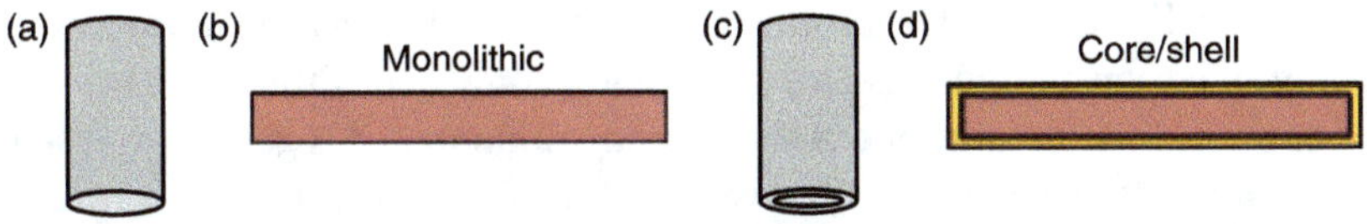

Figure 4.1 Schematic illustrations of the spinnerets used for, and products generated by, monoaxial and coaxial electrospinning. (a) A single-liquid spinneret for generating (b) monolithic fibres; (c) a coaxial spinneret, which results in (d) core/shell products.

delivering more complicated release profiles. Release can also be targeted to different parts of the body or particular cell types, and multifunctional fibres loaded with multiple active ingredients can be prepared. Proteins, which often degrade in single-liquid spinning owing to their fragile three-dimensional structures, can be processed, as can cells. Each of these will be discussed in turn below. In addition, as mentioned in Chapter 2, the shape and morphology of an electrospun product also depend on the material properties. By varying the properties of the working material, the use of a coaxial spinneret also enables the formation of a variety of other structures, including bubbles, scaffolds and multilayered fibres and particles.[2] Scientists have further sought to add additional liquids to the process, and we will finish the chapter with a discussion of three-liquid (triaxial) and four-liquid (quad-axial) processes.

4.2 Experimental considerations

The experimental set-up required for coaxial spinning was introduced in Chapter 2 (section 2.6). As for single-liquid spinning, to achieve a successful outcome it is necessary to consider carefully the properties of the solution and the processing parameters in the coaxial setting. The major considerations are the same as for single-liquid spinning (see section 3.2), but there are additional factors to take into account with coaxial spinning.

4.2.1 Handling two liquids

There are two fluid interfaces in the coaxial set-up: the liquid–gas interface between the sheath solution and the surrounding air, and the liquid–liquid interface between the two working solutions. Optimisation of the fluid interfaces is key in the formation of a stable compound cone jet, which in turn is critical for achieving uniform and reproducible core–shell products. The properties of the two solutions being processed cannot be considered in isolation. Although only one of the liquids (most commonly the sheath) needs to be electrospinnable, it is generally easier to achieve stable coflow if the two liquids have a relatively similar rate of solidification. If they do not, then there is a risk of one solution evaporating much faster than the other. This can cause clogging of the needle, and/or result in the separation of the two liquids. In turn, this leads to the properties of the fibres changing as a function of time during spinning, or separation of the core and shell fibre parts.

The charge distribution in a coaxial electrospinning jet is dependent on the properties of the core and sheath liquids. To form a cone shape as a compound droplet at the spinneret exit, at least one of the two liquids should enable a sufficient flow of charge. This is the driving liquid. In a typical monoaxial electrohydrodynamic process, the charge is localised at the interface between air and the charged liquid forming the Taylor cone. In a coaxial set-up, if the electrical relaxation time (time taken for an electron to travel in a material) of the sheath liquid is faster than or comparable to that of the core liquid, charges are localised at the outer interface between the sheath and the air, and the sheath liquid is the driving liquid. The core liquid can also act as the driving liquid if the outer is electrically insulating (a dielectric). In this case, when the driving interface is the inner one, the motion of the core liquid transmits to both the core and the sheath liquids via viscous force, setting the compound liquid in motion to form a coaxial jet.[3]

When the outermost sheath polymer solution has sufficient viscoelasticity, fibres with an encapsulated core are produced – this is coaxial electrospinning (or co-electrospinning). Hard-to-electrospin solutions or salts can be made into fibres by coaxial electrospinning, with a readily spinnable polymer serving as a template sheath for the core. If desired, the carrier polymer can be removed at a later stage. If the outermost sheath liquid does not allow sufficient molecular entanglement, coaxial electrospraying occurs, leading to core–shell particles.

As noted above, the integrity and reproducibility of the core–shell structure require simultaneous and concentric break-up of the compound jet. The relative behaviours of the two liquids will hence significantly impact the integrity of the core/shell structure in the fibres. The miscibility of the two liquids must be considered, as must volatility: a large difference between the boiling points of the solvents used can compromise the integrity of the core/shell structure generated during product solidification. Defects such as porous structures or molecules from the core leaching into the shell layer can arise if the core and shell solvents are miscible and evaporate at markedly different rates.[4] Careful consideration of the solvents available and optimisation of the interfacial compatibility are required in order to ensure the desired fibre products are generated.

The importance of flow rate has already been discussed in section 2.5.2; in coaxial spinning, the relative flow rates of the core and the shell liquids must also be considered. The faster the core flows with respect to the shell, the larger the core component of the fibres is expected to be. This tunability can be useful in varying the drug release profile, as will be discussed later. However, there is only a certain range of core-to-shell flow rate ratios over which the spinning process will be successful. At high core flow rates, there will not be a sufficiently fast rate of sheath solvent flow to encapsulate the core, leading to droplets with the two solutions mixed, or phase separation. The appropriate core-to-shell flow rate ratio is dependent on whether the core or the shell liquid is responsible for carrying the electrical charge (the driving liquid). Most commonly, when the shell liquid is the driver, a core-to-shell flow rate ratio of between around 1:3 and 1:10 is generally reported to give successful fibre formation, with lower ratios often (but not always) giving particles or mixtures of particles and fibres.[5] Higher ratios of 1:15 have also been reported to yield fibres successfully, however.[6] The exact range of ratios suitable for a particular experiment is dependent on the nature of the solutions used for the core and sheath, and needs investigation for each formulation being developed. The flow rate of the driving liquid carrying the charge also strongly affects the range of applied voltages that maintain the cone jet mode: higher flow rates of the driving liquid allow more charge to be carried per unit time and require a higher applied voltage to maintain a stable cone jet.

4.2.2 The spinneret and electrodes

The coaxial spinneret is conceptually simple, comprising one (narrower) needle nested inside another (Figure 4.1(c)). The exact diameters of the needles used can be varied, but in the authors' experience, we have had success using inner-needle internal diameters of 0.21–0.35 mm and an outer needle of 0.84–1.2 mm. Most researchers work with the ends of the two needles in line. However, the exact positions of the needles (does the inner needle protrude from the outer needle, and if so by how much, or vice versa?; Figure 4.2) can have an influence on the process, as illustrated by Sofokleous and co-workers.[7] These researchers found that having the inner needle displaced inside the outer needle by a small amount (2 mm in their systems) led to more homogeneous products and better encapsulation of the core inside the shell. Lee *et al.* have similarly developed what

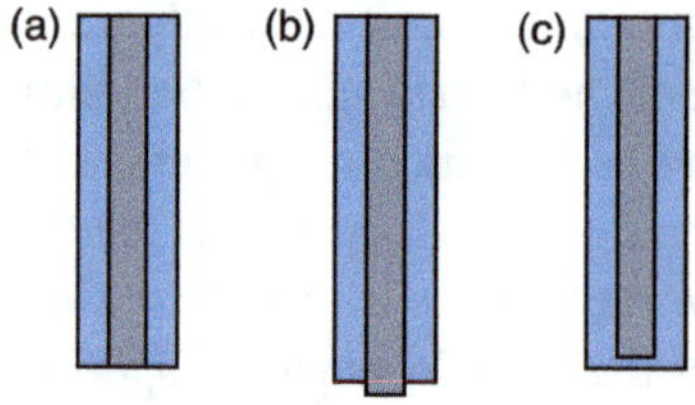

Figure 4.2 Possible needle configurations in coaxial electrospinning, showing (a) the inner and outer needles inline; (b) the inner needle protruding from the outer; and (c) the inner needle nested inside the outer.

they termed a 'core cut' nozzle where the terminus of the core needle is inside the shell needle, similar to Figure 4.2(c), and found that it reduced jet instability and gave more control over the spinning experiment.[8]

Most researchers use standard blunt-ended dispensing tips for electrospinning, but several studies suggest that covering the end of the needle with a plastic (e.g. Teflon or poly(vinyl chloride)) coating can be helpful. This is thought to reduce the attraction between the ejected polymer solution and the exterior of the needle, and can thereby reduce the formation of semi-solid substances on the syringe and the concomitant clogging which often arises.[9]

In the most common coaxial experiment, the spinneret is connected to the positive electrode of the high-voltage supply and the collector is connected to the negative electrode or grounded. Under a high electric field, the inner and outer liquids in the coaxial jet may separate or break into indistinct layers. This arises due to flow instability during the evaporation of solvent as the jet travels towards the collector. Practically, it is often difficult to stabilise a compound cone jet when the interfacial liquid properties are less than optimal. In this situation, the stability of the coaxial cone jet can be improved by the addition of grounded or negatively charged ring electrodes placed at specific distances away from positive coaxial spinneret positive polarity.[10] This approach has recently been proven powerful in coaxial electrospraying; since electrospraying and electrospinning differ only in the viscoelastic properties of the working liquids (see Chapter 2), improvements in the apparatus design and assembly for electrospray are usually applicable for electrospinning.

4.2.3 Establishing a coaxial process

The best place to start with developing a new process is to find a literature precedent which uses a similar polymer system. There exists a wealth of

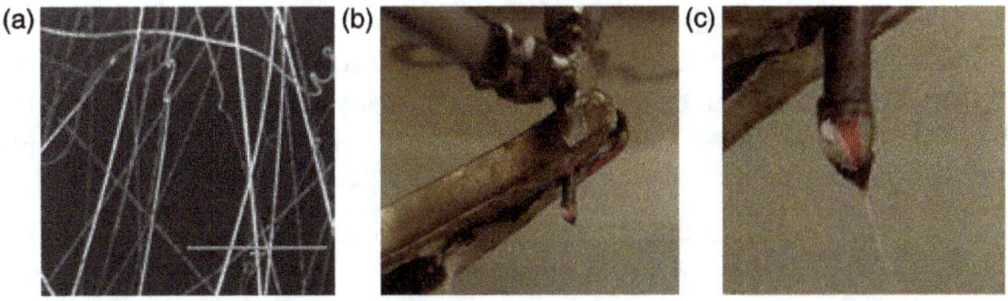

Figure 4.3 Optimising the fibre production process. (a) Fibres collected on a glass slide. Clear fibres can be seen, with no evidence for beads-on-string morphology. Some of the fibres are rather curved, however, which might be resolved by additional optimisation. Using a dye in the core liquid can aid visualisation of a coaxial process, as shown in (b) and enlarged in (c); a distinct two-liquid Taylor cone can be seen here, with the dye confined to the core liquid and no obvious liquid mixing. ((a) Courtesy of Alexandra Baskakova; (b and c) courtesy of Ukrit Angkawinitwong.)

information on single-liquid processes in particular, and thus a thorough review of the literature will likely reveal a protocol for a similar system to the one of interest. Using the closest possible literature parameters as a guide, we recommend initially spinning the two liquids singly and evaluating the fibres produced. If only one liquid in the process being developed is spinnable, then of course only this should be explored. The initial evaluation can be very crude, comprising simply collection of a few fibres (5–20 s of spinning or so) on a glass slide (or across a piece of cardboard with a hole cut in the middle) and holding them up to the light. If fibres have formed, this will be immediately obvious unless the fibres are below 400 nm in diameter. A more detailed assessment can then be undertaken by optical microscopy (Figure 4.3(a)).

Once fibres have been formed, a systematic variation in the voltage, spinneret-to-collector distance and flow rate for the single-liquid process is desirable, to observe which values give the best fibres. The products can be assessed by optical microscopy, and ideally will comprise fibres only with no particles/droplets. These fibres should possess uniform diameters, and no 'bead-on-string' morphologies should be visible. The optimisation process should be undertaken for each of the core and shell liquids. Coaxial electrospinning can then be commenced with the best set of parameters identified (or a compromise if very different parameters are found for the core and shell liquids).

In order to observe the behaviour of the liquids during initial coaxial experiments, it can be helpful to incorporate a small amount of a dye into the core liquid. This aids visualisation of the Taylor cone, and thus whether or not there is a compound cone with the core liquid nested neatly inside the shell can be established quickly (Figure 4.3(b) and (c)). Again, collection on to a glass slide or cardboard window will enable any fibres formed to be seen immediately, and can be followed by optical microscopy evaluations. If the dye is fluorescent, then in favourable instances (i.e. with large-diameter fibres) it will be possible to observe the core–shell structure using fluorescent light microscopy. Once the experimental parameters have been adjusted to obtain the best-quality fibres (see above) then the preparation of a larger-scale batch of fibres can commence. This should be followed by a detailed characterisation by scanning and transmission electron microscopy (SEM and TEM), X-ray diffraction, infrared spectroscopy, and so forth.

4.3 Extended-release systems

4.3.1 Preventing burst release

A standard approach to extending the time over which drug release from a polymer nanofibre occurs is to use a slow-dissolving or insoluble polymer in single-liquid spinning. However, a major problem which arises with single-liquid electrospinning is that, as a result of the very high surface-area-to-volume ratio of the fibres, a relatively large amount of the incorporated drug is present at or near the fibre surface. This commonly results in a *burst release*, where a significant proportion of the drug content is freed rapidly into solution at the start of the process.[4, 11] The initial burst is then usually followed by a tailing-off of the release rate. The burst release is not a problem when developing a fast-dissolving drug delivery system, because the aim is to release all the drug content into solution in a few seconds or minutes. It is, however, a major issue where modified-release systems are concerned.

The core/shell structures which can be obtained through coaxial electrospinning offer one potential solution to this issue. By preparing a two-compartment fibre, where the shell comprises a blank polymer and the drug is in the core alone, the problem of significant amounts of drug being present at the surface should be resolved if the shell polymer is insoluble or slow-dissolving. One of the first studies to investigate this possibility came from He and co-workers, who prepared fibres with a PLLA shell and a core comprising the antibiotic tetracycline hydrochloride (TCH) mixed with a low quantity of PLLA.[12] A small amount of a cross-linking agent was added to the shell solution to improve the mechanical

(a) (b)

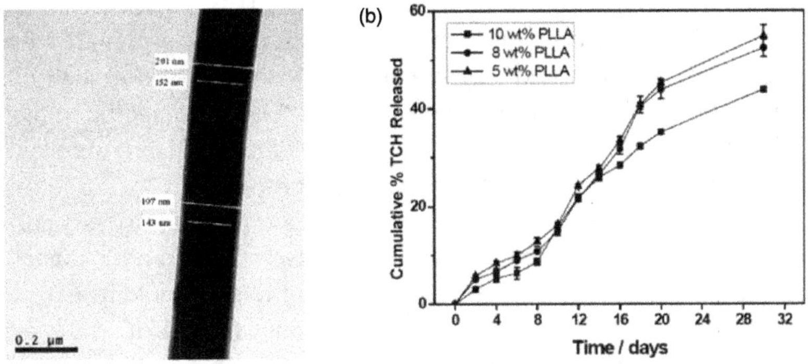

Figure 4.4 (a) Transmission electron microscopy image of a poly(L-lactic acid) (PLLA)/tetracycline hydrochloride (TCH) fibre prepared using a 10% w/v PLLA solution as the shell and a 5% w/v TCH/1% w/v PLLA core solution, and (b) TCH release from core/shell fibres prepared by He *et al.*[12] with the same TCH/PLLA core but varied concentrations of PLLA in the shell solution. (Adapted with permission from He, C. L.; Huang, Z. M.; Han, X. J.; Liu, L.; Zhang, H. S.; Chen, L. S. 'Coaxial electrospun poly(L-lactic acid) ultrafine fibers for sustained drug delivery.' *J. Macromol. Sci. B* 45 (2006): 515–524. Copyright Taylor & Francis 2006.)

properties and overcome the brittleness inherent to PLLA fibres. PLLA is a slow-degrading polymer (with a complete degradation time of more than 1 year under physiological conditions), and was employed because the aim of this work was to prepare antibacterial fibres for suturing or wound-dressing applications. TEM data showed the fibres to have clear core/shell structures (Figure 4.4(a)), and they were able to provide extended release over *ca.* 1 day. The production of core/shell systems in this work[12] additionally precluded the burst release previously reported from monolithic TCH-loaded fibres,[13] as shown in Figure 4.4(b).

Similar poly(lactic-co-glycolic acid) (PLGA) core/shell fibres, with both compartments made of PLGA and TCH in the core only, have been produced.[14] PLGA is another relatively slow-dissolving polymer (complete degradation time usually ≥ 2 months under physiological conditions), but despite this the fibres prepared showed a considerable burst release. The extent of the latter could be tuned by varying the polymer concentrations in the respective compartments, but it is clear that simply making a fibre with a shell of a slow-dissolving polymer and a drug-containing core does not necessarily prevent a burst release.

Coaxial electrospinning to produce fibres with TCH in the core has additionally been explored by Ramakrishna's team,[15] who prepared fibres with a PLGA (shell) and gum tragacanth (core). The core/shell fibres were found to be able to prolong the release period compared to monolithic fibres made from a blend of the two polymers, and also reduced the initial burst of release observed with the latter.

Analogous results have been seen for fibres comprising a poly(ε-caprolactone) (PCL) shell and a core of resveratrol (an antioxidant) or the antibiotic gentamicin sulfate, where drug release could be extended for more than 160 h.[16] PCL dissolves very slowly (over around 3 years *in vivo*), and thus these results are as intuitively expected. However, such findings are not ubiquitous. Hollow fibres were prepared consisting of a PCL shell with PEO and dexamethasone (an anti-inflammatory glucocorticoid) in the core, and despite the shell comprising PCL, a significant amount of burst release was observed.[17]

The observation that making fibres with a slow-dissolving shell does not necessarily prevent a burst release is well established in the literature. Such findings have been seen for systems with a polymer shell and drug-only core, for instance poly(L-lactide-co-ε-caprolactone) (PLCL) (shell)/heparin (core) fibres[18] and PLCL (shell)/paclitaxel (core) materials.[19] In both cases, despite the fact the drug was only present in the core, a notable burst release was seen.

A number of other authors have observed this phenomenon when using a drug/polymer matrix as the core solution rather than a simple drug solution, such as in the work of Zhu *et al.*[20] In this study, the authors used poly(lactic acid) (PLA), PCL or PLGA as the shell and a flurbiprofen axetil (non-steroidal anti-inflammatory drug)/poly(vinyl pyrrolidone) (PVP) blend for the core. Again, a large burst release was seen. The reasons behind such burst release are not entirely clear, since all of PLA, PLGA and PCL are slow to dissolve/degrade, but may arise as a result of some blending of the core and shell liquids, and/or the loaded drug being able to diffuse through pores in the shell.

The problem of burst release is particularly acute when working with hydrophilic active ingredients and biodegradable matrices, and Venkatraman's team have explored the use of coaxial spinning to ameliorate this issue.[21] Metoclopramide hydrochloride (MtpH; used for the treatment of nausea and vomiting) was used as a model active ingredient, and fibres prepared with PCL, PLLA and PLGA shells and a poly(vinyl alcohol) (PVA)/MtpH blend in the core. Significant amounts of burst release were observed with monolithic fibres spun from each of PCL, PLLA and PLGA. The coaxial PCL/PVA system reduced this burst somewhat, but a considerable amount of release was nevertheless observed in the first 6 h of dissolution testing. This was attributed to the presence of pores in the PCL shell. The coaxial PLLA/PVA and monolithic PLLA fibres behaved very similarly, which was believed to be because diffusion through the PLLA was the rate-limiting step to release, and the PLLA shell was not porous. The greatest difference in behaviour was observed with the PLGA systems, where the burst release was much suppressed in the coaxial fibres. In this instance, the rate of MtpH movement from the PVA core to the shell was the rate-determining step to release, and diffusion through the PLGA phase was relatively fast.

The work of Venkatraman *et al.* is important because it shows that merely making a core/shell fibre with drug located solely in the core and a slow-dissolving or insoluble shell is not sufficient to preclude burst release. It is important to consider the difference in hydrophilicity between the two polymers in the fibre; a moderate difference is required, because too great a difference may lead to a hollow core, as noted by Dror *et al.* (this arises because a very sharp interface forms between core and shell).[22] The drug itself needs to be more soluble in the core than the shell, and it is vital to control the electrospinning parameters to keep to a minimum the porosity of the shell (the ability of pores in a blank polymer shell to accelerate the rate of drug release from the core was also noted by Nguyen *et al.*[23]). Finally, the rate of drug diffusion through the shell needs to be considered: this should be relatively rapid, otherwise there is no benefit of using a core/shell system and no improvement in performance will be seen over a monolithic fibre of the shell polymer.

Zupančič *et al.* have built on these concepts, preparing fibres with an insoluble poly(methyl methacrylate) (PMMA) shell and a core of PVA or PVA/PMMA blends.[24] The core was loaded with the antibiotic ciprofloxacin, and the fibres proposed as advanced treatment modalities for a range of bacterial infections. The release rate could be tuned by varying the shell and core liquid flow rates and through the variation of the PMMA:PVA ratio in the core. In the optimal formulations, a burst release can be completely avoided and nearly zero-order release over a few days can be achieved (Figure 4.5).

A number of other studies have investigated drug-loaded core–shell fibres for extended release. For instance, a mixture of cellulose acetate (CA) and gelatin has been used to form the shell of a coaxial fibre loaded with the antibiotic amoxicillin and poly(ethylene glycol) (PEG) in the core.[25] Extended release over 1400 min was observed, with only a small burst release. However, it should be noted that the experiments were

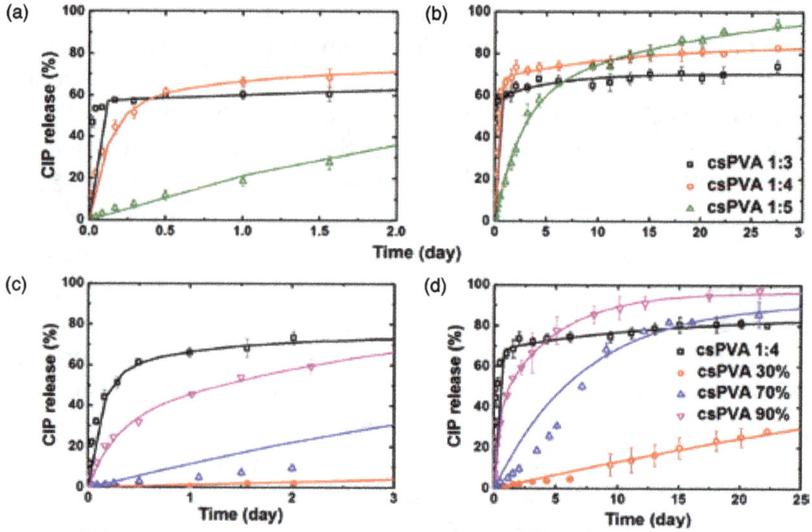

Figure 4.5 Tuning the rate of ciprofloxacin (CIP) release from core–shell poly(methyl methacrylate) (PMMA)/poly(vinyl alcohol) (PVA) fibers. (a) and (b) show the influence of varying the ratio of the core:shell flow rate from 1:3 to 1:5 in the preparation of PMMA (shell)/ PVA (core) (csPVA) systems. (c) and (d) depict the release profiles of fibres prepared at a 1:4 core:shell flow rate and with a PMMA/PVA blend core (percent values refer to the percentage of PVA in the core). (a) and (c) show the early stages of the release experiment, and (b) and (d) the full time period studied. (Adapted with permission from Zupančič, S.; Sinha-Ray, S.; Kristl, J.; Yarin, A. L. 'Controlled release of ciprofloxacin from core–shell nanofibers with monolithic or blended core.' *Mol. Pharm.* 13 (2016): 1393–1404. Copyright American Chemical Society 2016.)

conducted in a simulated gastric fluid at pH 1.2 throughout, not really representative of physiological conditions in the body.

In other work, Wang *et al.* have made core/shell PLLA/poly-(3-hydroxy butyrate) fibres with the enzyme inhibitor dimethyloxalylglycine in the core.[26] Again, by doing so they could make significant strides towards ameliorating burst release by localising the drug away from the release milieu.[26] Increasing the thickness of the fibre shell led to slower release in this work.

Further examples of coaxial electrospun core/shell fibres being exploited to reduce or preclude a burst release include those loaded with epidermal induction factors for skin regeneration,[27] the broad-spectrum antibiotic bacitracin,[28] the antiviral drug acyclovir,[29] silver nanoparticles for antibacterial applications,[30] dipyridamole to prevent platelet aggregation and reduce stroke risk[31] and tenofovir[32] or maraviroc[33] for anti-human immunodeficiency virus (HIV) treatment. The latter study employed ethyl cellulose (EC) as the shell and a PVP core, and found it was possible to tune the release rate by varying the shell thickness, with a thicker shell extending the release time. Similar results have been found with chitosan (shell)/PVA (core) fibres loaded with doxorubicin in the core,[34] and zein (shell)/zein-allyltriphenylphosphonium bromide (core) materials.[35]

There also exist reports of more sophisticated systems designed to sustain release and prevent the initial burst release. For instance, fibres have been prepared in which levofloxacin (an antibiotic) was first loaded on to mesoporous silica nanoparticles, and these in turn spun into the core of PCL fibres (with PCL comprising both the core and shell polymer).[36] A small reduction in burst release resulted from this system, and sustained release over more than 10 days was achieved. The use of the silica nanoparticles additionally extended the period of time over which the formulation was effective in preventing bacterial growth.

4.3.2 Biphasic release

Although it is commonly desirable to prevent a burst of release in the initial stages of dissolution, on occasion, and if it is properly controlled, such rapid release early on can be beneficial. This is because it can provide a *loading dose*, rapidly increasing the blood plasma concentration of drug into the therapeutic window. If a second, sustained, phase of release then ensues, a therapeutic concentration can be maintained over an extended period. This has been achieved on several occasions using core/shell electrospun fibres, and involves using an insoluble or slowly dissolving polymer as the core, and a fast-dissolving polymer for the shell. The drug is present in both phases. This concept has been demonstrated using the non-steroidal anti-inflammatory agent ketoprofen as a model drug, PVP as the shell polymer and either zein[37] or EC[38] as the core. When the fibres are added to the dissolution medium, the shell rapidly dissolves and frees its drug content into solution for the loading dose. The drug in the core is then released over a prolonged period of time. By varying the drug concentration in the different phases or the flow rates of the core and sheath liquids[38] it is possible to tune the amount of release in the first and second stages. Other work has used fibres with a CA shell and a core containing sodium hyaluronate and naproxen-loaded liposomes to achieve such a biphasic release profile.[39]

The above studies use a single-fibre formulation to deliver biphasic release, but it is also possible to achieve this by combining two different sets of fibres. Ball *et al.* have used this approach with core/shell fibres comprising an EC shell and PVP/maraviroc core.[33] Different fibres were prepared with varied shell/core thicknesses and then two formulations, one faster-releasing and one slow-releasing, physically mixed to provide a loading dose followed by sustained release of the remaining embedded drug.

4.4 Targeted drug delivery

Core/shell fibres generated by coaxial electrospinning have attracted attention for targeting the location of drug release in the body. In its simplest embodiment, this has taken the form of preparing fibres with the shell made of a pH-sensitive polymer (e.g. a Eudragit) which is insoluble at low pH. Such systems are designed for oral administration with the aim of preventing release in the stomach, where the shell is insoluble. Once the fibres enter the higher-pH lower parts of the intestine then the drug loading will be freed at a rate which can be controlled by judicious choice of the core polymer. For instance, fibres have been reported by Jin *et al.* in which the shell comprised Eudragit S100 (which dissolves at pH > 7) and the core made of PEO loaded with either gadolinium (III) diethylenetriaminepentaacetate hydrate or rhodamine B (Figure 4.6(a)).[40] The intention behind this work was to deliver an imaging agent locally to the colon for diagnosis of, for instance, irritable bowel syndrome. The authors found that the Eudragit coating successfully prevented almost all release in the pH conditions typical of the stomach, and upon an increase in pH to 7.4 (typical of the small intestine) the embedded functional ingredient was released in a sustained manner (Figure 4.6(b)). The imaging agents were unaffected by the electrospinning process, and were thus capable of imaging the colon, as was demonstrated *ex vivo* (Figure 4.6(c)). This approach was further extended to fibres loaded with both a drug and imaging agent for simultaneous imaging and drug delivery (so-called theranostic applications).[41]

However, as was noted for fibres designed to preclude a burst release, simply making core/shell materials with the exterior compartment made of a pH-sensitive polymer such as Eudragit will not necessarily result in the prevention of release in the stomach. Attempts to make such systems with 5-fluorouracil (5-FU; an anticancer drug) as

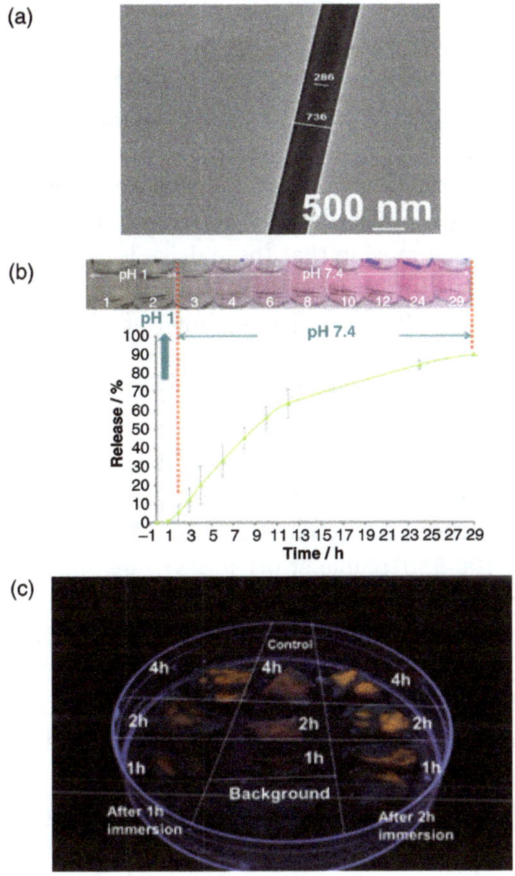

Figure 4.6 Data demonstrating the utility of core/shell poly(ethylene oxide)/Eudragit fibres loaded with rhodamine B in the core as colon-targeted imaging systems. (a) A transmission electron microscopy image of the fibres; (b) the rhodamine B release profile under varied pH conditions mimicking passage through the intestinal tract; (c) a photograph taken under ultraviolet light showing imaging of porcine colon by the fibres after they had been immersed in phosphate buffer to remove the Eudragit shell. The central column (control) is where a 50 ppm rhodamine B solution was added to the colon, while the left and right columns show results obtained after the fibres were placed in phosphate-buffered saline for 1 and 2 h, respectively, before being transferred to the colon sections. (Reproduced with permission from Jin, M.; Yu, D. G.; Wang, X.; Geraldes, C. F.; Williams, G. R.; Bligh, S. W. 'Electrospun contrast-agent-loaded fibers for colon-targeted MRI.' *Adv. Healthcare Mater.* 5 (2016): 977–985. Copyright John Wiley, 2016.)

the active ingredient failed, for example.[6] Fibres were generated with a blank Eudragit S100 shell and a drug-loaded core formed of PVP, EC, Eudragit S100 or drug alone. Clear core/shell morphology could be seen by TEM, yet in all cases significant amounts of release were seen at pH 1.0. This arose even though the drug was only present in the core, and the Eudragit sheath is insoluble at pH 1.0. The authors ascribe this to the low molecular weight of 5-FU and its relatively high solubility under acidic conditions, proposing that these drive it to diffuse through pores in the shell and escape into solution. The release profiles observed show an initial burst of release at pH 1.0, followed by a second burst when the pH is raised to 6.8. While these are potentially useful, they are not the colon-targeted profiles which the researchers hoped to achieve.

Similar results have been obtained by Yu and co-workers, although by design in this instance.[42] A Teflon-coated spinneret was employed here to aid the electrospinning process (see section 4.2.3 above), and fibres prepared with a Eudragit L100-55 (soluble at pH > 5.5) core and PVP sheath.[42] Helicid, an extract from Chinese herbal medicine commonly used to treat headaches and insomnia, was present in both parts of the fibre. The materials were shown to give an initial burst release (loading dose) of the drug at pH 2 (representative of the stomach), followed by sustained release at pH 7, as illustrated in Figure 4.7. This arises because the PVP exterior dissolves very rapidly at all pH conditions, freeing the drug in the shell. Further release at pH 2 is prevented because the core is insoluble, but once the pH is raised the core too becomes soluble and the remainder of the drug is freed.

Other researchers have adopted innovative ways in which electrospun core/shell systems can be used to target release. Zhou's group performed an elegant study in which they first synthesised a folate-conjugated PCL–PEG copolymer, then assembled this into micelles with the anticancer drug doxorubicin, and finally spun the micelles into the core of PVA (core)/gelatin (shell) fibres.[43] This was designed as an implantable device. The folate conjugation on the micelles enables them to target cancerous cells selectively, avoiding any damage to non-cancerous tissue. The systems were found to be able to release the doxorubicin incorporated over a prolonged period of time (> 100 h). During *in vivo* studies, application of the fibres directly to a tumour led to high local concentrations of the drug but low systemic levels, helpful in minimising side effects. Selective internalisation of the micelles to cancer cells was realised, ensuring low toxicity to normal tissue.

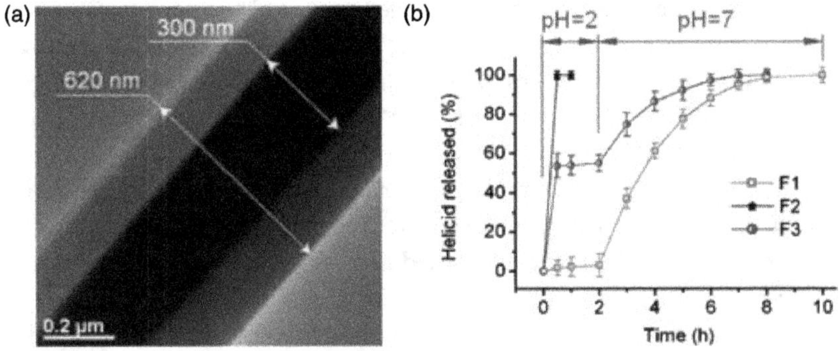

Figure 4.7 Using core/shell fibres to give targeted biphasic release. (a) Transmission electron microscopy image showing the two-compartment structure of poly(vinyl pyrrolidone) (PVP) (shell)/Eudragit L100-55 (core) systems with helicid loaded in both compartments. (b) Dissolution data for monolithic PVP/helicid (black) and Eudragit/helicid (green) fibres, together with the core/shell systems (blue). (Reproduced with permission from Yu, D.-G.; Liu, F.; Cui, L.; Liu, Z.-P.; Wang, X.; Bligh, S. W. A. 'Coaxial electrospinning using a concentric Teflon spinneret to prepare biphasic-release nanofibers of helicid.' *RSC Adv.* 3 (2013): 17775–17783. Copyright Royal Society of Chemistry, 2013.)

4.5 Multifunctional materials

The core/shell architecture of fibres from coaxial spinning naturally lends itself to the production of multifunctional materials, with different functional components loaded in the two compartments of the concentric structure. One of the earliest reports of this came from Ramakrishna's group, and explored the co-delivery of two model drugs, rhodamine B and bovine serum albumin (BSA) from PLCL fibres.[44] Electrospinning was performed using PLCL as the shell and a drug solution in the core, and the location of the two active ingredients was varied systematically. Unsurprisingly, the drug in the shell was released much more quickly than when incorporated in the core. An initial burst of release was seen in all cases, but this was reduced when the drug was loaded in the core of the matrix. Dual drug release systems have also been prepared in which vitamin C and E derivatives were encapsulated in the core of fibres with a poly(acrylonitrile) shell, with potential applications in the protection of skin from ultraviolet light.[45]

Another possibility is to incorporate additional excipients into the fibres. A flavour enhancer can be incorporated to mask the taste of bitter drugs, for example. Alternatively, surfactants could be added to solubilise poorly soluble active ingredients and/or enhance permeation through biomembranes. In one example of such work, fibres were prepared consisting of a PVP/acyclovir core and a PVP/sucralose/sodium dodecyl sulfate (DDS) shell.[46] Acyclovir is a potent systemic antiviral active ingredient, but suffers from poor solubility. In the fibres generated, it is present in the amorphous form, which leads to much faster dissolution than the pure drug powder. Sucralose is added as a sweetener to hide the metallic taste of the drug, and DDS acts as a permeation enhancer. As a result of the latter, increased permeation through the porcine sublingual mucosa (*cf.* the drug alone) was observed. The same approach of a PVP/sucralose shell and PVP/drug core has also successfully been implemented with helicid.[47] Similarly, PVP–quercetin/PVP–DDS core/shell fibres have been prepared.[48]

Multifunctional materials are of particular importance in tissue regeneration, and electrospun fibres have attracted some attention in this regard. Tang *et al.* prepared fibres with a core of PLGA/hydroxyapatite and a shell of collagen and amoxicillin.[49] The latter (an antibiotic) was intended to prevent infections occurring in wounds, and the core to promote bone growth. The drug release rate could be tuned by varying the collagen concentration in the shell liquid, and it was found that the core could effectively prevent the ingress of fibroblast cells, which is often an obstacle to successful bone regrowth.

For drugs which are acidic or basic (i.e. those which can donate or accept a proton), the pH at which dissolution happens will have a profound effect on solubility. Yan *et al.* have used core/shell fibres to enhance the solubility of quercetin, an acidic drug which is more soluble at elevated pHs.[50] Fibres were prepared with a PVP core containing quercetin and sodium hydroxide, and a shell of PVP and citric acid (Figure 4.8(a) and (b)). The components were all amorphously distributed in the polymer matrix, which exhibited much accelerated dissolution over the pure drug (Figure 4.8(c)). Inclusion of the NaOH in the core was believed to increase the solubility and dissolution rate of the drug since it would be ionised upon being freed from the fibres. This, combined with the amorphous nature of the drug in the formulation, raised the dissolution rate. Without the presence of the citric acid, the base in the core could have led to an increase in the pH of the dissolution medium (which *in vivo* would cause irritation or other side effects). The fact that an acid/base pair existed in the material, however, led to improved functional performance but no change to the pH of the medium.

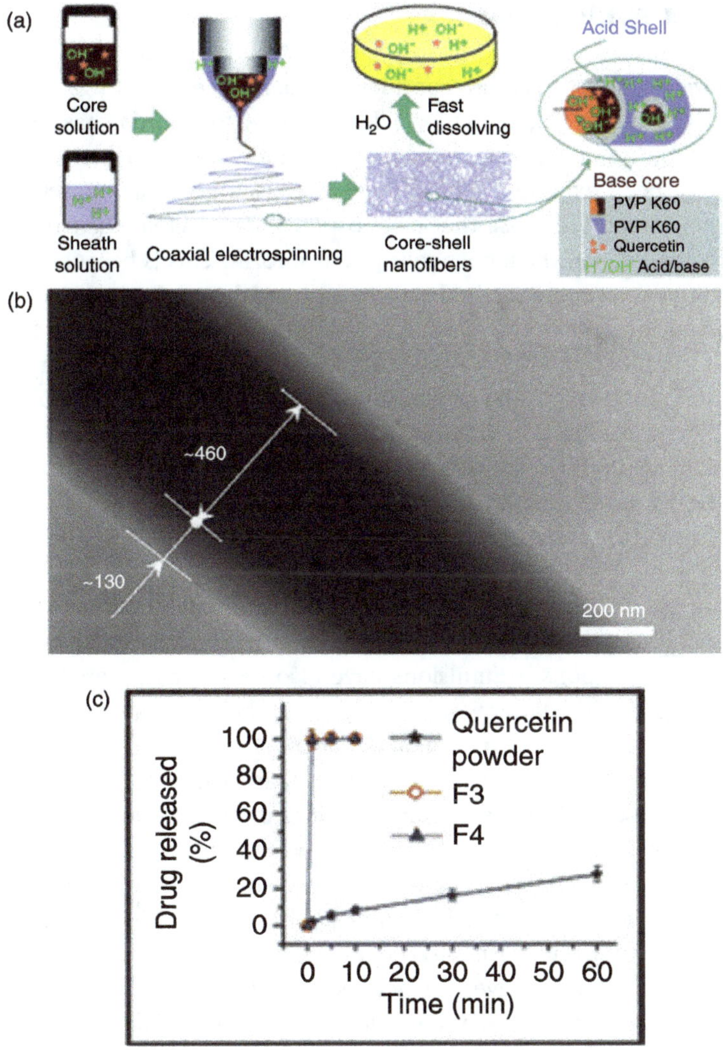

Figure 4.8 The preparation of acid–base pair solid dispersions using coaxial electrospinning. (a) A schematic of the approach used; (b) a transmission electron microscopy image of the core/shell poly(vinyl pyrrolidone) (PVP)–quercetin–NaOH/PVP–citric acid fibres; and (c) drug release data (F3 and F4 contain different amounts of quercetin). (Reproduced with permission from Yan, J.; Wu, Y.-H.; Yu, D.-G.; Williams, G. R.; Huang, S.-M.; Tao, W.; Sun, J.-Y. 'Electrospun acid–base pair solid dispersions of quercetin.' *RSC Adv.* 4 (2014): 58265–58271. Copyright Royal Society of Chemistry, 2014.)

4.6 Other applications

The above sections have all considered small-molecule drugs, and represent the major challenges to which coaxial electrospinning has been applied in this regard. There are additionally a few further applications which have been explored. As has been discussed previously (section 3.1), it is generally the case that electrospun fibres contain their functional components in the amorphous physical form. This is because the very fast solvent evaporation in the process causes the random molecular arrangement present in the starting solution to be propagated into the solid state, and because the polymer matrices in the fibres hinder recrystallisation. Dong's team have specifically looked at using core/shell fibres to prevent recrystallisation of the potent antimalarial drug artemisinin.[51] Conversion of the drug from the amorphous solid dispersion formed immediately after electrospinning to a crystalline material was found to be more rapid in monolithic blend fibres of PVP/CA/artemisinin than in coaxial systems with a PVP shell and CA/artemisinin core.

Core/shell fibres have been prepared with liposomes loaded in the core, in an attempt to ameliorate the stability issues which often plague liposomal formulations.[52] Emulsions have also been incorporated into the fibre core.[53] In the latter work by Viry *et al.*, the highly soluble drug levetiracetam (used for the treatment of epilepsy) was loaded into fibres with a PLGA solution acting as the shell liquid, and the core liquid comprising either a drug/PLGA solution or a water-in-oil emulsion with the drug in the dispersed aqueous droplets and the oil phase comprising a PLGA solution in dichloromethane. The emulsion fibres were able to extend the release time and reduce the amount of burst release seen at the early stages of the experiment.

Core/shell fibres have further been exploited for the self-assembly of magnetic chitosan nanoparticles with potential biomedical applications.[54] From fibres with a shell comprising PVP/chitosan and a core of PVP/Fe_3O_4 nanoparticles, Wang *et al.* were able to generate composite chitosan/Fe_3O_4 nanoparticles following addition of the fibres to acetone and drying.

4.7 Protein delivery systems

The small-molecule drugs discussed above can generally be processed by single-liquid electrospinning without problems, but it can be more desirable to prepare core/shell systems to deliver enhanced functional performance. In the case of proteins, however, coaxial electrospinning is often a requirement. This is because the activity of proteins is very dependent on their tertiary structure (a three-dimensional structure involving different parts of these large molecules being folded together and anchored by intermolecular forces such as hydrogen bonding). This tertiary structure is easily disrupted, leading to a loss of activity (denaturation), and once it is lost often cannot be regained. Given the need to use volatile solvents in single-liquid electrospinning and the propensity of these to denature proteins, the single-liquid process often cannot be used to prepare protein-loaded fibres with acceptable activity.[55] Further, the low solubility of many proteins in the non-aqueous solvents used in typical electrospinning processes means that only very low doses can be loaded.[55]

To resolve these problems, researchers have adopted two principal approaches. One is emulsion electrospinning, with protein-containing aqueous droplets distributed in a continuous phase, as discussed in section 3.11.1. The second is preparing core/shell systems by coaxial spinning. In such materials the core comprises a protein solution in a buffer designed to preserve the tertiary structure, possibly also containing stabilising excipients such as trehalose. The shell is a polymer solution in a volatile solvent.[55] The potency of this approach was first demonstrated by Jiang *et al.*, who used a PCL shell and a core of BSA or lysozyme and PEG.[56] PEG was included because it is known to help stabilise proteins. The proteins were found to be unaffected by the electrospinning process, and through variation of the flow rate of the core solution the protein release profile could be tuned. Similar results have been seen from an analogous system but with dextran used instead of PEG in the core.[57] Other proteins to have been explored in coaxial spinning include the enzyme lactose dehydrogenase[58] and gelatin.[59]

Romano *et al.* recently reported an elegant study in which they used the E-green fluorescent protein to investigate the electrospinning and release of a biological active ingredient from core/shell PEO/PCL fibres.[60] The photoluminescence spectrum of the fibres was virtually identical to the raw protein, indicating that the electrospinning process did not affect E-green fluorescent protein functionality (Figure 4.9). Release was observed to occur over an extended time period of more than 200 h.

The pH of the core protein solution has been proposed to be important in maintaining protein stability. Angkawinitwong *et al.* explored the effect of varying the pH of the core solution on the stability for bevacizumab (an antibody potent for the treatment of cancer and age-related degeneration in the eye).[61] Fibres were prepared with PCL as

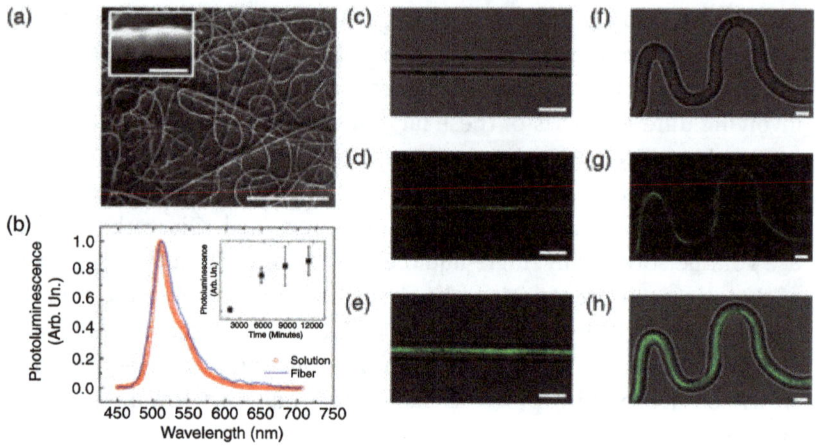

Figure 4.9 Data for core/shell PEO/PCL fibres loaded with E-green fluorescent protein (E-GFP). (a) Scanning electron microscopy image (scale bar: 100 μm) with enlargement of a single fibre in the inset (scale bar: 1 μm); (b) photoluminescence spectra of raw E-GFP in solution (red) and in the fibres (blue), with an inset showing the release of protein from the fibres; (c–h) confocal microscopy images (scale bars: 5 μm) of the fibres showing the transmission (c, f), fluorescence (d, g) and merged (e, h) images. (Reproduced with permission from Romano, L.; Camposeo, A.; Manco, R.; Moffa, M.; Pisignano, D. 'Core–shell electrospun fibers encapsulating chromophores or luminescent proteins for microscopically controlled molecular release.' *Mol. Pharm.* 13 (2016): 729–736. Copyright American Chemical Society 2016.)

the shell and a core solution buffered either to the isoelectric point (pI) of the protein (the pH at which it is neutral) or a pH below this. At the latter pH, the protein bore a net charge during electrospinning, which led to degradation. In contrast, the fibres fabricated at the pI ensured that the bevacizumab remained intact. They also permitted a constant rate of release to be maintained over 60 days.

A number of researchers have compared fibres from monoaxial and coaxial spinning. One such study produced fibres with a PCL shell and a core containing a fluorescently labelled BSA and compared these with those prepared in a blend electrospinning process.[62] The core/shell system was found able to reduce the initial burst release during *in vitro* dissolution experiments, as also observed for small-molecule-loaded core/shell fibres (see section 4.3.1). Also working with PCL, Jansen's team investigated the differences between single-liquid and coaxial spinning of BSA and alkaline phosphatase.[63] The core/shell systems both extended release for longer periods of time and proved better able to maintain the biological activity of the protein.

A similar study compared these two processes in the preparation of PLGA fibres loaded with fibroblast growth factor-2 (FGF-2), known to be important in tissue repair and stem cell proliferation and differentiation.[64] The protein encapsulation efficiency and release profiles were similar for both types of fibres, with the monolithic fibres from single-liquid spinning releasing the protein somewhat more rapidly, as would be expected. Bone marrow stem cells were cultured on the fibres, but no clear conclusions could be drawn as to the relative efficacy of the two spinning methodologies in this regard.

Chitosan has also been explored as a filament-forming matrix for FGF-2, with both emulsion and coaxial emulsion (i.e. either the core or shell liquid is an emulsion) spinning compared as delivery systems.[65] No intact growth factor could be found in the monolithic emulsion fibres. In the core/shell case, inclusion of FGF-2 into the core rather than the shell of the fibres led to the presence of more intact protein in the formulation, in addition to improved cell adhesion and spreading. FGF-2 has further been incorporated into PCL (shell)/PEO (core) fibres.[66] Sustained release of the active ingredient over more than 9 days was observed.

There are a number of additional studies investigating core/shell fibres for the delivery of growth factors. For instance, Kong's group prepared materials with a PLCL shell and a core comprising dextran and platelet-derived growth factor-BB.[67] Smooth-muscle cells were cultured with the fibres, which were found to promote cell attachment and increase cellular activity.

In other work, nerve growth factor (NGF) has been incorporated into the core of PLCL shell fibres.[68] These materials were explored *in vivo* in rats, and found to have potential in promoting nerve regrowth.[68a] Similar fibres have been produced with PLA shells and silk fibroin cores loaded with NGF, and reported to aid the growth of the elongated neurite cells required for nerve growth.[69] Some authors have sought to prepare more sophisticated systems, in which the concentration of the NGF was varied through the thickness of the fibre mat.[70] The shell of the fibres comprised PCL, with a PEG/BSA/NGF core (BSA was added as a carrier protein and to help stabilise the NGF). A peristaltic pump was used to vary the NGF concentration in the solution used for spinning, such that the initial fibres collected contained a different NGF content to those collected at the end of the experiment. The side of the mat formed of fibres with the higher NGF concentration led to a higher percentage of cells having neurite outgrowths. Sustained release of both NGF and BSA was seen.

Core-shell fibres with PLGA shells and PVA/transforming growth factor-β (TGF-β) cores have been produced and compared with monolithic blend PLGA/PVA/TGF-β fibres.[71] The core/shell fibres had potential in directing stem cell differentiation for the treatment of spinal injuries, and led to slower release of the loaded growth factor than the monolithic fibres. However, over the timescale studied they were less effective in promoting differentiation than the monolithic analogues.

Vascular endothelial growth factor (VEGF) has also been incorporated into fibres with a PLGA shell and a dextran/BSA/heparin/VEGF core.[72] VEGF was freed from the fibres over more than 25 days, with only a small burst release noted. Cells could spread effectively on the fibres, which additionally did not cause any undesirable immune response. Seyednejad *et al.* have further explored a mixture of the polyester poly(hydroxymethylglycolide-co-ε-caprolactone) and PCL as the shell and VEGF/BSA as the core.[73] The addition of the polyester helped to accelerate protein release, which is likely to be desirable since PCL degrades very slowly in the body (over 2–4 years). Again, the VEGF was found to retain its biological activity post-electrospinning.

Multiple bioactive factors may be incorporated into a single fibre, as demonstrated by Chen's group for TGF-β and stem cell affinity peptide E7.[74] TGF-β was loaded in the core of PCL (shell)/PVP-BSA (core) fibres, and the peptide subsequently covalently bound to the exterior. The presence of the peptide promoted the initial adhesion of stem cells, while the TGF-β was freed from the matrices over around 20 days, maintaining its bioactivity throughout this time and promoting the differentiation of stem cells into cartilage cells. Such scaffolds hence have significant potential for connective tissue engineering.

Shalumon and co-workers have developed multifunctional growth factor-loaded fibres for bone regrowth.[75] Their materials consisted of a silk fibroin/chitosan shell loaded with nanosized hydroxyapatite particles, and bone morphogenetic protein-2 in the core. The release of protein from the core aided the differentiation of stem cells into osteoblasts and the presence of hydroxyapatite in the shell helped to direct bone growth. PLGA (shell)/collagen (core) fibres co-loaded with fibronectin and cadherin 11 – biomolecules known to be important in bone growth and cell adhesion – have additionally been reported.[76]

Other types of biomolecules which have been processed using coaxial electrospinning include a model virus,[77] which was incorporated into the core of PCL (shell)/PEG (core) fibres. These were found to release the virus over more than 2 weeks, and the released virus was determined to be less immunogenic than the unprocessed virus. These materials could have great potential in the development of viral gene delivery systems for a range of applications where defective DNA needs to be corrected, for instance in cystic fibrosis or severe combined immune deficiency. Non-viral genes can also be delivered through the coaxial electrospinning technology. For instance, plasmid DNA has been incorporated into the core of coaxial electrospun fibres.[78] A gene delivery vector was loaded into the shell of the fibres, which were shown to act as extended-release systems potent in cell transfection over a prolonged period of time.

4.8 Cell electrospinning

Beyond proteins and other small biomolecules, researchers have also found it is possible to process living cells through coaxial electrospinning. This field of research has been pioneered by Jayasinghe, with the first report in 2006.[79] A suspension of human 1321N1 astrocytoma (brain tumour) cells in culture medium at a concentration of 10^6 cells mL^{-1} was used as the core liquid, with a poly(dimethylsiloxane) solution as the sheath. No statistical differences were observed between cell viability post-electrospinning and of control cells passed through a needle but without any potential difference applied. Follow-on work demonstrated that it is possible to process cells at very high concentrations of up to 10^7 per mL.[80]

Cell-loaded fibre mats have successfully been grafted into mice, and the ability of the cells to proliferate *in vivo* was found to be unaffected by the electrospinning process.[81] A range of cell types has been electrospun, with a number of resultant applications. For instance, cardiac myocytes have been spun into fibres with potential application in cardiac tissue engineering.[82]

In order to ensure that the cells remain viable post-spinning, the collector used for cell electrospinning needs to be considered carefully, and differs from the metal plates or cylinders most commonly employed. Collection is usually into a Petri dish or other container filled with a cell culture medium, with a grounded ring electrode placed above or below this. If required, a wire mesh can be inserted into the medium to provide a structure on which a scaffold can be constructed. Experiments are also usually performed in a laminar flow hood to ensure sterility. The apparatus commonly used is depicted in Figure 4.10, together with an image of electrospun cardiac cells.[82] It should also be noted that the polymers used for cell electrospinning must be highly biocompatible in order to

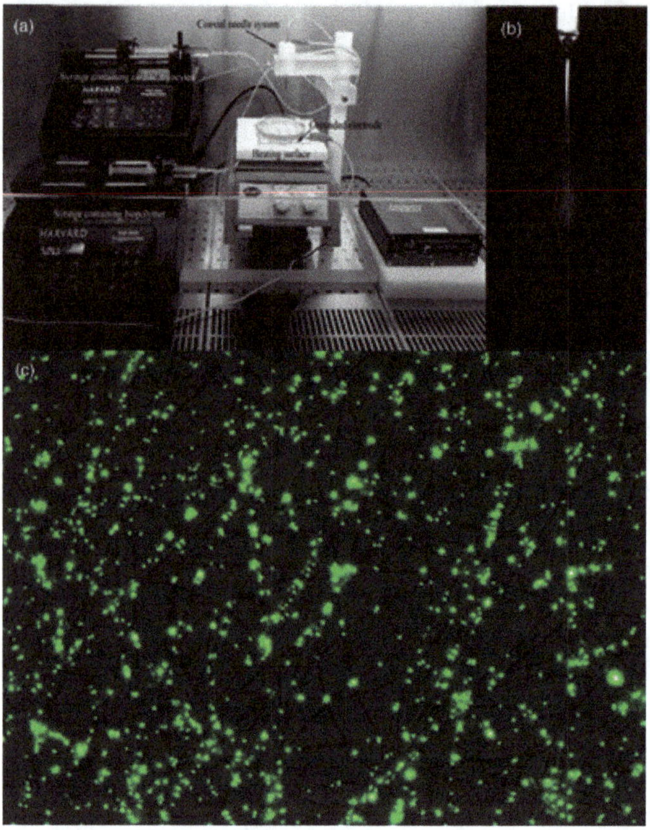

Figure 4.10 Cell electrospinning. (a) The experimental set-up; (b) a photograph taken during the spinning process; and (c) a combined bright-field and fluorescence image of the cell-loaded electrospun scaffold. The cells can be seen in green and the fibre meshes in black. (Reproduced with permission from Ehler, E.; Jayasinghe, S. N. 'Cell electrospinning cardiac patches for tissue engineering the heart.' *Analyst* 139 (2014): 4449–4452. Copyright Royal Society of Chemistry 2014.)

maximise viability. This, and other, detailed experimental considerations are discussed in some recent reviews.[83]

4.9 Modified coaxial spinning

As discussed above, it was initially thought that for successful coaxial electrospinning a spinnable shell solution was required, while the core liquid did not necessarily need to be processable alone by electrospinning. However, this is not always the case, and it turns out that a wide variety of non-spinnable shell solutions can be processed too. This can be achieved if the core liquid is a spinnable polymer solution,[84] or even a common solvent without a carrier polymer.[85] Working with an unspinnable shell solution has been termed *modified coaxial electrospinning* in the literature. It was first reported by Han and Steckl in 2009,[84] with the first application of the technique in drug delivery following in 2010.[86] The latter employed a pure solvent or solvent mixture as the sheath liquid, and very concentrated solutions of the PVP or Eudragit L100 polymers as the core, yielding monolithic fibres from a two-liquid process. Coaxial electrospinning was successful even when the core polymer solution was too concentrated to be electrospun in the standard single-liquid set-up.

This work was built upon to explore the influence of the shell solvent on the fibre properties (morphology, diameter, etc.), and the modified coaxial products were found to have reduced diameters and greater diameter homogeneity compared to analogous materials from single-liquid spinning.[87] A shell liquid comprising LiCl in *N,N*-dimethylacetamide (DMAc) has also been shown to be able to reduce the diameter of poly(acrylonitrile) (PAN) fibres, giving materials with smoother surfaces and reduced polydispersity.[88] The presence of a blank solvent or solvent blend outside the polymer core is believed to perform a number of functions, including reducing surface tension at the exit to the spinneret and slowing down the evaporation of the core solvent (by replacing the air/polymer solution interface with a solvent/solution interface).[89] This in turn can be helpful in preventing the formation of solid substances on the spinneret and subsequent blocking of the working liquid flow,[90] and hence it is possible to run spinning processes for much longer without manual intervention. Surfactant solutions can be used to similar ends.[91]

Such processes are of interest for drug delivery applications, because they offer new ways to tailor the arrangement of components in the fibres, and in particular the possibility of preparing in one step a polymer fibre with a functionalised exterior. For instance, using a solution of $AgNO_3$ as the sheath liquid and a PAN core solution, PAN fibres with $AgNO_3$ at the surface can be prepared.[92] Exposing these to ultraviolet light reduces the $AgNO_3$ to Ag nanoparticles, resulting in highly effective antibacterial materials. The benefit of the modified coaxial approach over the single-liquid monoaxial process is that it allows a functional ingredient to be localised at the surface; in this particular example, such localisation is very useful because any Ag trapped inside the fibres would have no efficacy. By ensuring the Ag nanoparticles are only at the surface, there is no wasted material, which is beneficial in both cost and environmental terms. It is also possible to use a solution of a hydrophobic molecule such as stearic acid as the sheath, resulting in polymer fibres with a hydrophobic coating; this has been reported to improve the stability to humidity of PVP fibres, which usually are extremely hygroscopic.[93]

A direct comparison of ketoprofen-loaded CA fibres prepared by single-liquid electrospinning and those generated in a modified coaxial process with a mixture of DMAc, acetone and ethanol as the sheath liquid has been undertaken.[94] The modified coaxial fibres were found to be narrower and less polydisperse in their diameters than those from the single-liquid experiment, as shown in Figure 4.11(a)–(f). Both sets of fibres contained the drug in the amorphous physical form, and the dissolution profiles were similar (Figure 4.11(g)). However, the modified coaxial fibres showed more linear release between 8 and 144 h, and reached a higher overall release percentage. This indicates that the use of the sheath solvent has promise in preparing high-quality drug delivery systems.

Similar observations have been reported for zein/ibuprofen fibres,[95] and for Eudragit L100/sodium diclofenac materials using both blank solvent[96] and a salt solution as the shell.[97] A further study explored the preparation of fibres comprising CA and ferulic acid (an antioxidant commonly found in Chinese traditional herbal medicine), with PVP as an additional component.[98] The use of a blank sheath solvent reduced fibre diameter and improved polydispersity as before, and the inclusion of PVP helped to control the rate of drug release and ameliorate the problem of 'tailing off' (a slowing down in the release rate) which often arises with monolithic formulations. Analogous results were reported for systems comprising PAN/PVP and ibuprofen prepared using the modified set-up.[99]

Fibres prepared through the modified coaxial route have been explored as a template for self-assembly of solid lipid nanoparticles.[100] Materials were produced using PVP, tristearin and naproxen. Increasing the flow rate of the ethanol solvent used as the sheath liquid caused a reduction in the diameter of the composite fibres. When the fibres were added to water, the tristearin and naproxen spontaneously self-assembled into nanoparticles (see section 3.13), with narrower fibres resulting in smaller particles. These could play an important role in enhancing permeation through biomembranes, although no drug release or permeation studies of the self-assembled particles were reported.

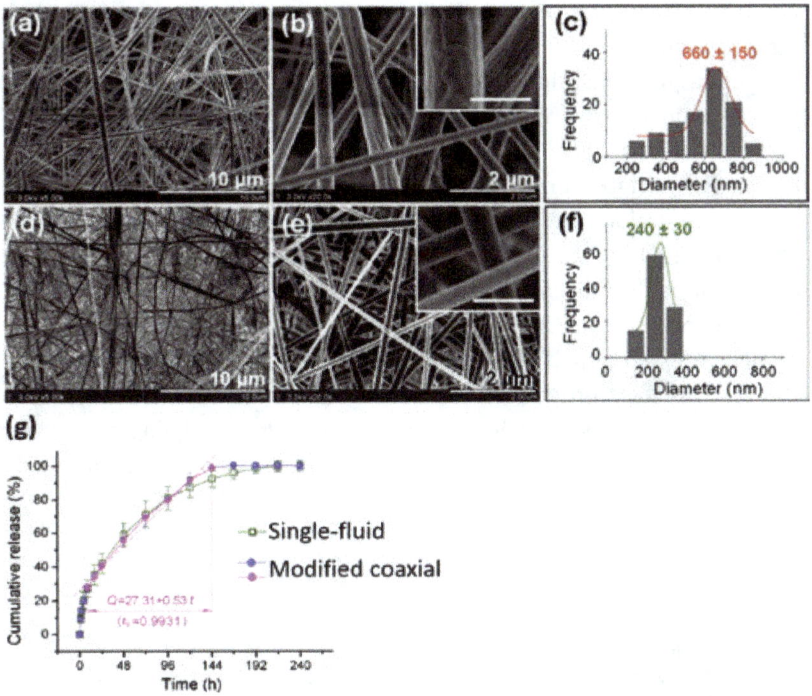

Figure 4.11 A comparison of ketoprofen-loaded cellulose acetate fibres prepared by single-liquid and modified coaxial electrospinning. (a–c) Surface morphologies and diameter distribution of single-liquid fibres; (d–f) surface morphologies and diameter distribution of modified coaxial fibres; (g) dissolution profiles of the two sets of fibres. The scale bars in the insets of (b) and (e) represent 500 nm. (Reproduced from Yu, D. G.; Yu, J. H.; Chen, L.; Williams, G. R.; Wang, X. 'Modified coaxial electrospinning for the preparation of high-quality ketoprofen-loaded cellulose acetate nanofibers.' *Carbohydr. Polym.* 90 (2012): 1016–1023, with permission from Elsevier. Copyright Elsevier 2012.)

Biphasic release formulations have additionally been prepared from modified coaxial spinning. Here, the sheath solution is not a blank solvent or salt solution, but rather an unspinnable polymer solution. In one example of such work, Li *et al.* generated fibres using a spinnable EC/quercetin solution as the core and an unspinnable PVP/quercetin shell.[9b] They also used a poly(vinyl chloride) coating for the spinneret to aid the spinning process (see section 4.2.3 above). The products comprised core/shell fibres (Figure 4.12(a)). The PVP shell dissolved very rapidly to release a loading dose of drug, while the EC core then gave sustained release. The amount of release in the first phase could be controlled by varying the drug content in the shell (Figure 4.12(b)). Similar findings have been noted with paracetamol as the active ingredient.[101]

Formulations with close to zero-order release have been prepared from modified coaxial spinning.[102] Experiments were undertaken with an unspinnable low-concentration CA shell solution and a spinnable higher-concentration CA/ketoprofen core. This led to fibres with a drug-loaded core and a shell of CA alone. The CA shell was able to ameliorate the burst release observed from analogous monolithic CA/ketoprofen materials, and thus provide a release profile close to being zero-order over 96 h. This approach has additionally been demonstrated for zein/ketoprofen systems.[103]

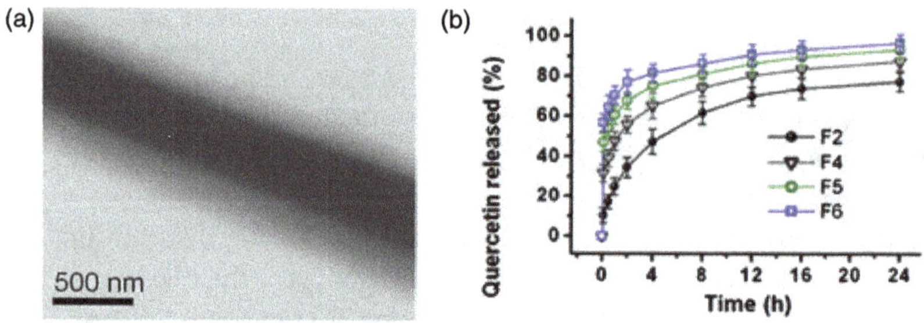

Figure 4.12 Core/shell ethyl cellulose (EC)/poly(vinyl pyrrolidone) (PVP) fibres loaded with quercetin prepared by modified coaxial electrospinning. A series of fibres was prepared; formulation F2 comprises EC/quercetin fibres from single-liquid spinning, while F4–F6 are core/shell EC/PVP systems generated through the modified coaxial experiment, with increasing amounts of quercetin in the shell. (a) Transmission electron microscopy image of F5, showing the two-component architecture. (b) The results of dissolution testing, showing that increasing the amount of drug in the fibres leads to an increase in the percentage of release in the initial burst phase. (Adapted with permission from Li, C.; Wang, Z.-H.; Yu, D.-G.; Williams, G. R. 'Tunable biphasic drug release from ethyl cellulose nanofibers fabricated using a modified coaxial electrospinning process.' *Nanoscale Res. Lett.* 9 (2014): 258.)

4.10 Triaxial and quad-axial systems

To produce high-quality multi-compartment fibres, it is necessary to ensure that there is no merging between the spinning solutions. This means either the compartmentalised solutions need to be immiscible or all the solutions need to lose solvent at similar rates: if one of the liquids dries faster than the others, then separation of the different compartments may arise. The first reports of triaxial electrospinning emerged from Lallave and co-workers[104] in 2007 and Kalra *et al.* in 2009.[105] The former report is concerned with using the resultant fibres to generate carbon nanotubes. The latter authors used silica in the core and outer layers. The middle layer comprised a block copolymer mixed with either magnetite nanoparticles or a second polymer, with the aim of making self-assembled structures in the confined space between the silica layers. Triaxial spinning has also been used to tune and optimise the mechanical properties of polystyrene/polyurethane-containing fibres.[106]

The earliest example of a triaxial drug delivery system emerged from the work of Han and Steckl, who made fibres containing PVP and PCL loaded with two dyes as model drug molecules (Figure 4.13).[107] The authors were aiming to overcome the problem of burst release that can arise with core/shell fibres if the shell is made of a hygroscopic (and therefore fast-dissolving) material. A hygroscopic shell is often desirable, however, in order to impart the fibres with good biocompatibility properties. A three-layer system with a drug-loaded core, hydrophobic middle layer and hygroscopic outer layer can combine both of these benefits (Figure 4.13).

In Han and Steckl's work, they made some progress towards their goal by developing triaxial electrospinning and preparing materials with a hydrophobic exterior. Fibres were made with a core comprising PVP, and the middle and outer layers consisting of PCL.[107] Two different dyes were incorporated, one in the core and one in the outer layer. The latter dye was released very rapidly, while sustained release from the core was seen. By varying the dimensions of the inner, middle and outer needles in the spinneret, it was possible to modulate the rate of release from the PVP core, while the dye in the shell was freed similarly rapidly in all cases.

Yu and co-workers, mindful of the need for the liquids being processed in triaxial spinning to have similar properties, have generated three-layer fibres from three solutions of EC containing varying concentrations of ketoprofen, a non-steroidal anti-inflammatory drug.[108] The different concentrations of ketoprofen in each of the three

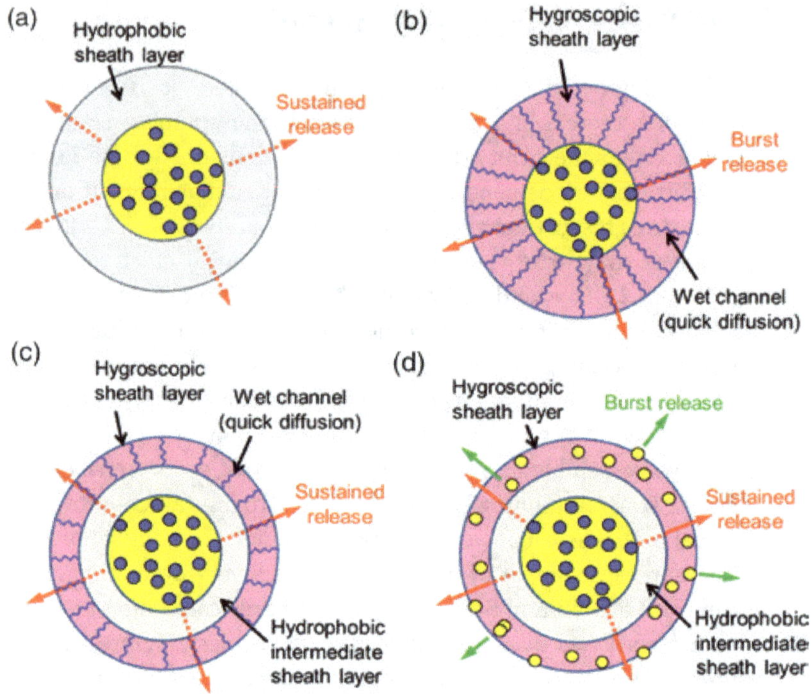

Figure 4.13 Schematic showing the benefits of using triaxial electrospinning to prepare fibres which have a hygroscopic shell while preventing burst release of the incorporated drug. (a) A coaxial fibre with a hydrophobic shell will show sustained release, but may have poor biocompatibility, while (b) such a fibre with a hygroscopic shell will lead to rapid drug release, often obviating any benefits of the core/shell structure. (c) A triaxial system with a hygroscopic sheath can both give sustained release and ensure biocompatibility. (d) Drug could also be loaded into the outer layer of the fibres to deliver a loading dose. (Reproduced with permission from Han, D.; Steckl, A. J. 'Triaxial electrospun nanofiber membranes for controlled dual release of functional molecules.' *ACS Appl. Mater. Interfaces* 5 (2013): 8241–8245. Copyright American Chemical Society 2013.)

solutions resulted in fibres with a gradient distribution of the drug. The concentration of drug increased moving from the shell of the systems inwards. TEM images show that the fibres have a clear trilayer structure (Figure 4.14(a)), with all the components having the amorphous physical form.

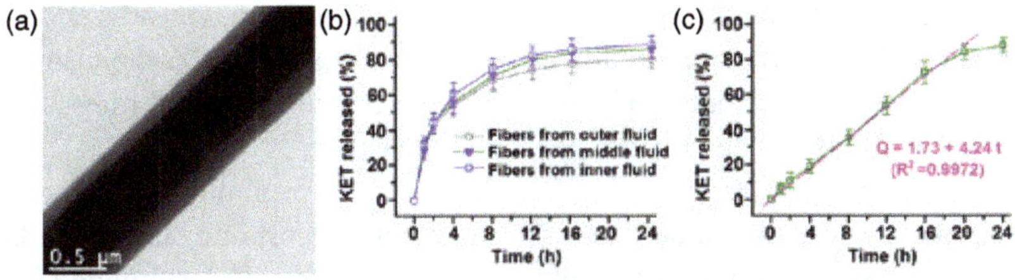

Figure 4.14 Data on the three-layer ethyl cellulose/ketoprofen (KET) fibres prepared by Yu *et al.* (a) A transmission electron microscopy image showing the internal structure of the systems; (b) the KET release profiles from monolithic fibres generated from each of the individual spinning solutions with different drug loadings; (c) the zero-order KET release profile of the three-layer fibres. (Reproduced with permission from Yu, D. G.; Li, X. Y.; Wang, X.; Yang, J. H.; Bligh, S. W.; Williams, G. R. 'Nanofibers fabricated using triaxial electrospinning as zero order drug delivery systems.' *ACS Appl. Mater. Interfaces* 7 (2015): 18891–18897. Copyright American Chemical Society 2015.)

As has been discussed previously, a major drawback with monolithic fibres is the initial burst of drug release which is typically seen. When monolithic fibres were prepared from the individual EC/ketoprofen solutions with different drug concentrations, such burst release was indeed observed (Figure 4.14(b)). The release profiles are virtually identical, regardless of the drug loading in the fibres. However, the three-layer fibres from triaxial spinning were found to give zero-order release over around 20 h, with a constant rate of drug release throughout this time (Figure 4.14(c)).

This release profile was realised by balancing three key factors. EC is insoluble in water, and thus drug release from this system will be controlled by the rate at which the ketoprofen molecules can diffuse out of the polymer matrix. Drug molecules in the shell of the fibre are very close to the dissolution medium and thus do not have to diffuse far to reach the solution. The shell also has the largest surface area of the three compartments. The ketoprofen molecules in the middle layer have to diffuse further to reach the outside of the fibres, and this layer also has a smaller surface area. If the drug concentration were the same in both the shell and middle layers, there would be more rapid drug release from the former. However, the increase in drug concentration going from the shell to the middle compartment compensates both for the increased diffusion distance and reduced surface area, leading to both compartments having the same release rate. The same considerations apply to the core: again, the increased drug concentration compensates for the greater distance the ketoprofen molecules must travel to escape from the fibres and the further reduced surface area.

One of the major benefits of multi-axial electrospinning is that non-spinnable solutions can be processed so long as at least one of the liquids being processed is spinnable on its own. This has been well documented for coaxial electrospinning, and although less explored, initial reports suggest it is equally true for triaxial spinning.[109] Yang *et al.* successfully prepared fibres using a modified triaxial process in which the outer liquid was pure ethanol, the middle liquid a solution of Eudragit S100 and the core liquid a solution of lecithin and diclofenac sodium. Only the middle liquid here is individually spinnable, and the authors hence propose that a triaxial process can be undertaken with only one spinnable liquid so long as the two non-spinnable ones are not in contact.[109] The Eudragit/lecithin/diclofenac fibres were found to act as pH-sensitive drug delivery systems, with the Eudragit precluding release at acidic pH. At neutral pH, diclofenac was released in a novel two-stage process. Some drug was freed directly into solution upon dissolution of the Eudragit, but the majority of the drug and lecithin initially combined to form hydrophobic nanoparticles. These subsequently freed the embedded diclofenac, leading to both sustained release and increased permeation through the intestinal mucosa.

The modified triaxial approach has further been applied to prepare nanoscale drug depot fibres.[110] A solvent sheath liquid was employed to surround a CA middle layer, which in turn encompassed a core comprising a ferulic acid solution. This led to a system where partially crystalline ferulic acid was trapped inside a CA-based fibre. The release rate of the drug was controlled by its rate of diffusion through the CA, which resulted in close to zero-order release over around 36 h. These fibres showed reduced initial burst and tailing-off effects compared to monolithic CA/ferulic acid materials prepared from modified coaxial spinning. The drug depot fibres could not be prepared directly in coaxial electrospinning, because rapid solidification of the shell CA led to blocking of the spinneret.

Given the paucity of reports on three-liquid electrospinning, it is not surprising that relatively little work has been done to explore the effect of the processing parameters on the success of the process. However, some detail is known on the effect of solvent volatility and polymer molecular weight for systems of PCL and CA.[111] Fibres were prepared with a CA shell, PCL intermediate layer and a mineral oil core. The latter was then removed by dissolution in octanol to produce hollow materials. It was found that for successful electrospinning it was important to have the outer working liquid composed of a more volatile solvent system than the middle liquid, and also for the molecular weight of the outer polymer to be greater than or equal to that of the middle polymer.

There are only a few reports of triaxial spinning in the literature so far. This is most likely due to the difficulty in equilibrating the multiple liquid interfaces and the rate of solvent evaporation in a concentric jetting process with three or more coflowing liquids. On the other hand, there has been much effort in generating multilayered particles via triaxial and multi-axial electrospraying, the sister technique of electrospinning. As described in Chapter 2, electrospraying and electrospinning use the same set-up and differ only in the viscoelastic properties of the working liquids, which are primarily determined by the polymer concentrations and molecular chain length. The solvent choices that are optimal for coaxial and multi-axial electrospray could be helpful for optimising solvent choices and the handling of multiple liquids in coaxial and multi-axial electrospinning. Interested readers are directed to Chapter 6, section 6.8, for discussions on electrospraying.

It is possible in principle to process four, five or even more liquids: the complexity of such processes increases rapidly with the number of liquids being processed, however, which explains why only one report of a four-fluid electrospinning process could be found in the literature.[112] In this work, Labbaf *et al.* used a four-needle (quad-axial) spinneret and electrospun four-layer core/shell fibres made of different biocompatible polymers: PEG, PLGA, PCL and poly(methylsilsesquioxane). The multilayered four-liquid electrospinning technique has significant potential in drug delivery applications, however, as it offers the advantages of achieving in one formulation the delivery of multiple active pharmaceutical ingredients in a time-dependent fashion as demanded by the course of treatment.

4.11 Conclusions

This chapter has introduced the concept of coaxial electrospinning, and provided some details on how to implement the experiment. We have then discussed the various ways in which the approach has been applied to drug delivery, including the prevention or reduction of burst release, giving biphasic or targeted release and preparing multi-functional materials. Its utility in processing more complex active biomolecules such as proteins, and even cells, has been considered, as has the modified coaxial electrospinning process where only the core is spinnable. Finally, the possibilities of triaxial and quad-axial spinning and the layered materials it can produce have been enumerated. Overall, it is clear that multi-axial electrospinning offers the ability to generate increasingly complicated nano- and micro-scale architectures, with concomitantly enhanced functional performance. The caveat is that the experiment becomes increasingly complex as the number of liquids being processed increases; this is particularly important when consideration is given to scaling up the process. We will return to this topic in Chapter 7.

4.12 References

1. Sun, Z.; Zussman, E.; Yarin, A. L.; Wendorff, J. H.; Greiner, A. 'Compound core–shell polymer nanofibers by co-electrospinning.' *Adv. Mater.* 15 (2003): 1929–1931.
2. (a) Ahmad, Z.; Zhang, H. B.; Farook, U.; Edirisinghe, M.; Stride, E.; Colombo, P. 'Generation of multilayered structures for biomedical applications using a novel tri-needle coaxial device and electrohydrodynamic flow.' *J. R. Soc. Interface.* 5 (2008): 1255–1261; (b) Ekemen, Z.; Ahmad, Z.; Stride, E.; Kaplan, D.; Edirisinghe, M. 'Electrohydrodynamic bubbling: An alternative route to fabricate porous structures of silk fibroin based materials.' *Biomacromolecules* 14 (2013): 1412–1422.
3. (a) Diaz, J. E.; Barrero, A.; Marquez, M.; Loscertales, I. G. 'Controlled encapsulation of hydrophobic liquids in hydrophilic polymer nanofibers by co-electrospinning.' *Adv. Funct. Mater.* 16 (2006): 2110–2116; (b) Loscertales, I. G.; Barrero, A.; Guerrero, I.; Cortijo, R.; Marquez, M.; Ganan-Calvo, A. M. 'Micro/nano encapsulation via electrified coaxial liquid jets.' *Science* 295 (2002): 1695–1698.
4. Chou, S. F.; Carson, D.; Woodrow, K. A. 'Current strategies for sustaining drug release from electrospun nanofibers.' *J. Control. Release* 220 (2015): 584–591.
5. Chakraborty, S.; Liao, I. C.; Adler, A.; Leong, K. W. 'Electrohydrodynamics: A facile technique to fabricate drug delivery systems.' *Adv. Drug Deliv. Rev.* 61 (2009): 1043–1054.
6. Illangakoon, U. E.; Yu, D. G.; Ahmad, B. S.; Chatterton, N. P.; Williams, G. R. '5-Fluorouracil loaded Eudragit fibers prepared by electrospinning.' *Int. J. Pharm.* 495 (2015): 895–902.
7. Sofokleous, P.; Lau, W. K.; Edirisinghe, M.; Stride, E. 'The effect of needle tip displacement in co-axial electrohydrodynamic processing.' *RSC Adv.* 6 (2016): 75258–75268.
8. Lee, B. S.; Jeon, S. Y.; Park, H.; Lee, G.; Yang, H. S.; Yu, W. R. 'New electrospinning nozzle to reduce jet instability and its application to manufacture of multi-layered nanofibers.' *Sci. Rep.* 4 (2014): 6758.

9. (a) Xiang, Q.; Ma, Y.-M.; Yu, D.-G.; Jin, M.; Williams, G. R. 'Electrospinning using a Teflon-coated spinneret.' *Appl. Surf. Sci.* 284 (2013): 889–893; (b) Li, C.; Wang, Z.-H.; Yu, D.-G.; Williams, G. R. 'Tunable biphasic drug release from ethyl cellulose nanofibers fabricated using a modified coaxial electrospinning process.' *Nanoscale Res. Lett.* 9 (2014): 258.
10. Zhang, L.; Si, T.; Fischer, A. J.; Letson, A.; Yuan, S.; Roberts, C. J.; Xu, R. X. 'Coaxial electrospray of ranibizumab-loaded microparticles for sustained release of anti-VEGF therapies.' *PLoS ONE* 10 (2015): e0135608.
11. (a) Zupančič, Š.; Baumgartner, S.; Lavrič, Z.; Petelin, M.; Kristl, J. 'Local delivery of resveratrol using polycaprolactone nanofibers for treatment of periodontal disease.' *J. Drug Del. Sci. Technol.* 30 (2015): 408–416; (b) Sebe, I.; Szabo, P.; Kallai-Szabo, B.; Zelko, R. 'Incorporating small molecules or biologics into nanofibers for optimized drug release: A review.' *Int. J. Pharm.* 494 (2015): 516–530; (c) Pelipenko, J.; Kocbek, P.; Kristl, J. 'Critical attributes of nanofibers: Preparation, drug loading, and tissue regeneration.' *Int. J. Pharm.* 484 (2015): 57–74.
12. He, C. L.; Huang, Z. M.; Han, X. J.; Liu, L.; Zhang, H. S.; Chen, L. S. 'Coaxial electrospun poly(L-lactic acid) ultrafine fibers for sustained drug delivery.' *J. Macromol. Sci. B* 45 (2006): 515–524.
13. Kenawy, E.-R.; Bowlin, G. L.; Mansfield, K.; Layman, J.; Simpson, D. G.; Sanders, E. H.; Wnek, G. E. 'Release of tetracycline hydrochloride from electrospun poly(ethylene-co-vinylacetate), poly(lactic acid), and a blend.' *J. Control. Release* 81 (2002): 57–64.
14. Maleki, M.; Latifi, M.; Amani-Tehran, M.; Mathur, S. 'Electrospun core–shell nanofibers for drug encapsulation and sustained release.' *Polym. Eng. Sci.* 53 (2013): 1770–1779.
15. Ranjbar-Mohammadi, M.; Zamani, M.; Prabhakaran, M. P.; Bahrami, S. H.; Ramakrishna, S. 'Electrospinning of PLGA/gum tragacanth nanofibers containing tetracycline hydrochloride for periodontal regeneration.' *Mater. Sci. Eng. C* 58 (2016): 521–531.
16. Huang, Z. M.; He, C. L.; Yang, A.; Zhang, Y.; Han, X. J.; Yin, J.; Wu, Q. 'Encapsulating drugs in biodegradable ultrafine fibers through co-axial electrospinning.' *J. Biomed. Mater. Res. A* 77 (2006): 169–179.
17. Rubert, M.; Li, Y.-F.; Dehli, J.; Taskin, M. B.; Besenbacher, F.; Chen, M. 'Dexamethasone encapsulated coaxial electrospun PCL/PEO hollow microfibers for inflammation regulation.' *RSC Adv.* 4 (2014): 51537–51543.
18. Su, Y.; Li, X.; Liu, Y.; Su, Q.; Qiang, M. L.; Mo, X. 'Encapsulation and controlled release of heparin from electrospun poly(L-lactide-co-epsilon-caprolactone) nanofibers.' *J. Biomater. Sci. Polym. Ed.* 22 (2011): 165–177.
19. Huang, H. H.; He, C. L.; Wang, H. S.; Mo, X. M. 'Preparation of core–shell biodegradable microfibers for long-term drug delivery.' *J. Biomed. Mater. Res. A* 90 (2009): 1243–1251.
20. Zhu, T.; Yang, C.; Chen, S.; Li, W.; Lou, J.; Wang, J. 'A facile approach to prepare shell/core nanofibers for drug controlled release.' *Mater. Lett.* 150 (2015): 52–54.

21. Tiwari, S. K.; Tzezana, R.; Zussman, E.; Venkatraman, S. S. 'Optimizing partition-controlled drug release from electrospun core–shell fibers.' *Int. J. Pharm.* 392 (2010): 209–217.
22. Dror, Y.; Kuhn, J.; Avrahami, R.; Zussman, E. 'Encapsulation of enzymes in biodegradable tubular structures.' *Macromolecules* 41 (2008): 4187–4192.
23. Nguyen, T. T.; Ghosh, C.; Hwang, S. G.; Chanunpanich, N.; Park, J. S. 'Porous core/sheath composite nanofibers fabricated by coaxial electrospinning as a potential mat for drug release system.' *Int. J. Pharm.* 439 (2012): 296–306.
24. Zupančič, S.; Sinha-Ray, S.; Kristl, J.; Yarin, A. L. 'Controlled release of ciprofloxacin from core–shell nanofibers with monolithic or blended core.' *Mol. Pharm.* 13 (2016): 1393–1404.
25. Kiatyongchai, T.; Wongsasulak, S.; Yoovidhya, T. 'Coaxial electrospinning and release characteristics of cellulose acetate–gelatin blend encapsulating a model drug.' *J. Appl. Polym. Sci.* 131 (2014): 40167.
26. Wang, C.; Yan, K.-W.; Lin, Y.-D.; Hsieh, P. C. H. 'Biodegradable core/shell fibers by coaxial electrospinning: Processing, fiber characterization, and its application in sustained drug release.' *Macromolecules* 43 (2010): 6389–6397.
27. Jin, G.; Prabhakaran, M. P.; Kai, D.; Ramakrishna, S. 'Controlled release of multiple epidermal induction factors through core-shell nanofibers for skin regeneration.' *Eur. J. Pharm. Biopharm.* 85 (2013): 689–698.
28. Yao, J.; Zhang, S.; Li, W.; Du, Z.; Li, Y. '*In vitro* drug controlled-release behavior of an electrospun modified poly(lactic acid)/bacitracin drug delivery system.' *RSC Adv.* 6 (2016): 515–521.
29. Azizi, M.; Seyed Dorraji, M. S.; Rasoulifard, M. H. 'Influence of structure on release profile of acyclovir loaded polyurethane nanofibers: Monolithic and core/shell structures.' *J. Appl. Polym. Sci.* 133 (2016): 44073.
30. Khodkar, F.; Golshan Ebrahimi, N. 'Preparation and properties of antibacterial, biocompatible core–shell fibers produced by coaxial electrospinning.' *J. Appl. Polym. Sci.* 134 (2017): 44979.
31. Repanas, A.; Glasmacher, B. 'Dipyridamole embedded in polycaprolactone fibers prepared by coaxial electrospinning as a novel drug delivery system.' *J. Drug Del. Sci. Technol.* 29 (2015): 132–142.
32. Meng, J.; Agrahari, V.; Ezoulin, M. J.; Zhang, C.; Purohit, S. S.; Molteni, A.; Dim, D.; Oyler, N. A.; Youan, B. C. 'Tenofovir containing thiolated chitosan core/shell nanofibers: *In vitro* and *in vivo* evaluations.' *Mol. Pharm.* 13 (2016): 4129–4140.
33. Ball, C.; Chou, S. F.; Jiang, Y.; Woodrow, K. A. 'Coaxially electrospun fiber-based microbicides facilitate broadly tunable release of maraviroc.' *Mater. Sci. Eng. C* 63 (2016): 117–124.
34. Yan, E.; Fan, Y.; Sun, Z.; Gao, J.; Hao, X.; Pei, S.; Wang, C.; Sun, L.; Zhang, D. 'Biocompatible core–shell electrospun nanofibers as potential application for chemotherapy against ovary cancer.' *Mater. Sci. Eng. C* 41 (2014): 217–223.

35. Li, J.; Feng, H.; He, J.; Li, C.; Mao, X.; Xie, D.; Ao, N.; Chu, B. 'Coaxial electrospun zein nanofibrous membrane for sustained release.' *J. Biomater. Sci. Polym. Ed.* 24 (2013): 1923–1934.
36. Jalvandi, J.; White, M.; Truong, Y. B.; Gao, Y.; Padhye, R.; Kyratzis, I. L. 'Release and antimicrobial activity of levofloxacin from composite mats of poly(εcaprolactone) and mesoporous silica nanoparticles fabricated by core–shell electrospinning.' *J. Mater. Sci.* 50 (2015): 7967–7974.
37. Jiang, Y. N.; Mo, H. Y.; Yu, D. G. 'Electrospun drug-loaded core–sheath PVP/zein nanofibers for biphasic drug release.' *Int. J. Pharm.* 438 (2012): 232–239.
38. Yu, D. G.; Wang, X.; Li, X. Y.; Chian, W.; Li, Y.; Liao, Y. Z. 'Electrospun biphasic drug release polyvinylpyrrolidone/ethyl cellulose core/sheath nanofibers.' *Acta Biomater.* 9 (2013): 5665–5672.
39. Li, Z.; Kang, H.; Che, N.; Liu, Z.; Li, P.; Li, W.; Zhang, C.; Cao, C.; Liu, R.; Huang, Y. 'Controlled release of liposome-encapsulated naproxen from core–sheath electrospun nanofibers.' *Carbohydr. Polym.* 111 (2014): 18–24.
40. Jin, M.; Yu, D. G.; Wang, X.; Geraldes, C. F.; Williams, G. R.; Bligh, S. W. 'Electrospun contrast-agent-loaded fibers for colon-targeted MRI.' *Adv. Healthcare Mater.* 5 (2016): 977–985.
41. Jin, M.; Yu, D. G.; Geraldes, C. F.; Williams, G. R.; Bligh, S. W. 'Theranostic fibers for simultaneous imaging and drug delivery.' *Mol. Pharm.* 13 (2016): 2457–2465.
42. Yu, D.-G.; Liu, F.; Cui, L.; Liu, Z.-P.; Wang, X.; Bligh, S. W. A. 'Coaxial electrospinning using a concentric Teflon spinneret to prepare biphasic-release nanofibers of helicid.' *RSC Adv.* 3 (2013): 17775–17783.
43. Yang, G.; Wang, J.; Wang, Y.; Li, L.; Guo, X.; Zhou, S. 'An implantable active-targeting micelle-in-nanofiber device for efficient and safe cancer therapy.' *ACS Nano* 9 (2015): 1161–1174.
44. Su, Y.; Su, Q.; Liu, W.; Jin, G.; Mo, X.; Ramakrishna, S. 'Dual-drug encapsulation and release from core–shell nanofibers.' *J. Biomater. Sci. Polym. Ed.* 23 (2012): 861–871.
45. Wu, X. M.; Branford-White, C. J.; Yu, D. G.; Chatterton, N. P.; Zhu, L. M. 'Preparation of core–shell PAN nanofibers encapsulated alpha-tocopherol acetate and ascorbic acid 2-phosphate for photoprotection.' *Colloids Surf. B* 82 (2011): 247–252.
46. Yu, D. G.; Zhu, L. M.; Branford-White, C. J.; Yang, J. H.; Wang, X.; Li, Y.; Qian, W. 'Solid dispersions in the form of electrospun core–sheath nanofibers.' *Int. J. Nanomedicine* 6 (2011): 3271–3280.
47. Wu, Y.-H.; Yu, D.-G.; Li, X.-Y.; Diao, A.-H.; Illangakoon, U. E.; Williams, G. R. 'Fast-dissolving sweet sedative nanofiber membranes.' *J. Mater. Sci.* 50 (2015): 3604–3613.
48. Li, X. Y.; Li, Y. C.; Yu, D. G.; Liao, Y. Z.; Wang, X. 'Fast disintegrating quercetin-loaded drug delivery systems fabricated using coaxial electrospinning.' *Int. J. Mol. Sci.* 14 (2013): 21647–21659.

49. Tang, Y.; Chen, L.; Zhao, K.; Wu, Z.; Wang, Y.; Tan, Q. 'Fabrication of PLGA/HA (core)–collagen/amoxicillin (shell) nanofiber membranes through coaxial electrospinning for guided tissue regeneration.' *Compos. Sci. Technol.* 125 (2016): 100–107.
50. Yan, J.; Wu, Y.-H.; Yu, D.-G.; Williams, G. R.; Huang, S.-M.; Tao, W.; Sun, J.-Y. 'Electrospun acid–base pair solid dispersions of quercetin.' *RSC Adv.* 4 (2014): 58265–58271.
51. Shi, Y.; Zhang, J.; Xu, S.; Dong, A. 'Electrospinning of artemisinin-loaded core–shell fibers for inhibiting drug re-crystallization.' *J. Biomater. Sci. Polym. Ed.* 24 (2013): 551–564.
52. Li, Z.; Kang, H.; Li, Q.; Che, N.; Liu, Z.; Li, P.; Zhang, C.; Liu, R.; Huang, Y. 'Ultrathin core–sheath fibers for liposome stabilization.' *Colloids Surf. B* 122 (2014): 630–637.
53. Viry, L.; Moulton, S. E.; Romeo, T.; Suhr, C.; Mawad, D.; Cook, M.; Wallace, G. G. 'Emulsion-coaxial electrospinning: Designing novel architectures for sustained release of highly soluble low molecular weight drugs.' *J. Mater. Chem.* 22 (2012): 11347–11353.
54. Wang, B.; Zhang, P.-P.; Williams, G. R.; Branford-White, C.; Quan, J.; Nie, H.-L.; Zhu, L.-M. 'A simple route to form magnetic chitosan nanoparticles from coaxial-electrospun composite nanofibers.' *J. Mater. Sci.* 48 (2013): 3991–3998.
55. Jiang, H.; Wang, L.; Zhu, K. 'Coaxial electrospinning for encapsulation and controlled release of fragile water-soluble bioactive agents.' *J. Control. Release* 193 (2014): 296–303.
56. Jiang, H.; Hu, Y.; Li, Y.; Zhao, P.; Zhu, K.; Chen, W. 'A facile technique to prepare biodegradable coaxial electrospun nanofibers for controlled release of bioactive agents.' *J. Control. Release* 108 (2005): 237–243.
57. Jiang, H.; Hu, Y.; Zhao, P.; Li, Y.; Zhu, K. 'Modulation of protein release from biodegradable core–shell structured fibers prepared by coaxial electrospinning.' *J. Biomed. Mater. Res. B* (2006): 50–57.
58. Moreno, I.; González-González, V.; Romero-García, J. 'Control release of lactate dehydrogenase encapsulated in poly (vinyl alcohol) nanofibers via electrospinning.' *Eur. Polym. J.* 47 (2011): 1264–1272.
59. Sakuldao, S.; Yoovidhya, T.; Wongsasulak, S. 'Coaxial electrospinning and sustained release properties of gelatin–cellulose acetate core–shell ultrafine fibre.' *ScienceAsia* 37 (2011): 335–343.
60. Romano, L.; Camposeo, A.; Manco, R.; Moffa, M.; Pisignano, D. 'Core–shell electrospun fibers encapsulating chromophores or luminescent proteins for microscopically controlled molecular release.' *Mol. Pharm.* 13 (2016): 729–736.
61. Angkawinitwong, U.; Awwad, S.; Khaw, P. T.; Brocchini, S.; Williams, G. R. 'Electrospun formulations of bevacizumab for sustained release in the eye.' *Acta Biomater.* 64 (2017): 126–136.
62. Zhang, Y. Z.; Wang, X.; Feng, Y.; Lim, C. T.; Ramakrishna, S. 'Coaxial electrospinning of (fluorescein isothiocyanate-conjugated bovine serum

albumin)-encapsulated poly(E-caprolactone) nanofibers for sustained release.' *Biomacromolecules* 7 (2006): 1049–1057.

63. Ji, W.; Yang, F.; van den Beucken, J. J.; Bian, Z.; Fan, M.; Chen, Z.; Jansen, J. A. 'Fibrous scaffolds loaded with protein prepared by blend or coaxial electrospinning.' *Acta Biomater.* 6 (2010): 4199–4207.
64. Sahoo, S.; Ang, L. T.; Goh, J. C.; Toh, S. L. 'Growth factor delivery through electrospun nanofibers in scaffolds for tissue engineering applications.' *J. Biomed. Mater. Res. A* 93 (2010): 1539–1550.
65. Place, L. W.; Sekyi, M.; Taussig, J.; Kipper, M. J. 'Two-phase electrospinning to incorporate polyelectrolyte complexes and growth factors into electrospun chitosan nanofibers.' *Macromol. Biosci.* 16 (2016): 371–380.
66. Rubert, M.; Dehli, J.; Li, Y.-F.; Taskin, M. B.; Xu, R.; Besenbacher, F.; Chen, M. 'Electrospun PCL/PEO coaxial fibers for basic fibroblast growth factor delivery.' *J. Mater. Chem. B* 2 (2014): 8538–8546.
67. Li, H.; Zhao, C.; Wang, Z.; Zhang, H.; Yuan, X.; Kong, D. 'Controlled release of PDGF-bb by coaxial electrospun dextran/poly(L-lactide-co-epsilon-caprolactone) fibers with an ultrafine core/shell structure.' *J. Biomater. Sci. Polym. Ed.* 21 (2010): 803–819.
68. (a) Liu, J. J.; Wang, C. Y.; Wang, J. G.; Ruan, H. J.; Fan, C. Y. 'Peripheral nerve regeneration using composite poly(lactic acid-caprolactone)/nerve growth factor conduits prepared by coaxial electrospinning.' *J. Biomed. Mater. Res. A* 96 (2011): 13–20; (b) Yan, S.; Xiaoqiang, L.; Lianjiang, T.; Chen, H.; Xiumei, M. 'Poly(L-lactide-co-ε-caprolactone) electrospun nanofibers for encapsulating and sustained releasing proteins.' *Polymer* 50 (2009): 4212–4219.
69. Tian, L.; Prabhakaran, M. P.; Hu, J.; Chen, M.; Besenbacher, F.; Ramakrishna, S. 'Coaxial electrospun poly(lactic acid)/silk fibroin nanofibers incorporated with nerve growth factor support the differentiation of neuronal stem cells.' *RSC Adv.* 5 (2015): 49838–49848.
70. Handarmin; Tan, G. J.; Sundaray, B.; Marcy, G. T.; Goh, E. L.; Chew, S. Y. 'Nanofibrous scaffold with incorporated protein gradient for directing neurite outgrowth.' *Drug Deliv. Transl. Res.* 1 (2011): 147–160.
71. Cui, X.; Liu, M.; Wang, J.; Zhou, Y.; Xiang, Q. 'Electrospun scaffold containing TGF-beta1 promotes human mesenchymal stem cell differentiation towards a nucleus pulposus-like phenotype under hypoxia.' *IET Nanobiotechnol.* 9 (2015): 76–84.
72. Jia, X.; Zhao, C.; Li, P.; Zhang, H.; Huang, Y.; Li, H.; Fan, J.; Feng, W.; Yuan, X.; Fan, Y. 'Sustained release of VEGF by coaxial electrospun dextran/PLGA fibrous membranes in vascular tissue engineering.' *J. Biomater. Sci. Polym. Ed.* 22 (2011): 1811–1827.
73. Seyednejad, H.; Ji, W.; Yang, F.; van Nostrum, C. F.; Vermonden, T.; van den Beucken, J. J.; Dhert, W. J.; Hennink, W. E.; Jansen, J. A. 'Coaxially electrospun scaffolds based on hydroxyl-functionalized poly(epsilon-caprolactone) and loaded with VEGF for tissue engineering applications.' *Biomacromolecules* 13 (2012): 3650–3560.

74. Man, Z.; Yin, L.; Shao, Z.; Zhang, X.; Hu, X.; Zhu, J.; Dai, L.; Huang, H.; Yuan, L.; Zhou, C.; Chen, H.; Ao, Y. 'The effects of co-delivery of BMSC-affinity peptide and rhTGF-beta1 from coaxial electrospun scaffolds on chondrogenic differentiation.' *Biomaterials* 35 (2014): 5250–5260.
75. Shalumon, K. T.; Lai, G. J.; Chen, C. H.; Chen, J. P. 'Modulation of bone-specific tissue regeneration by incorporating bone morphogenetic protein and controlling the shell thickness of silk fibroin/chitosan/nanohydroxyapatite core–shell nanofibrous membranes.' *ACS Appl. Mater. Interfaces* 7 (2015): 21170–21181.
76. Wang, J.; Cui, X.; Zhou, Y.; Xiang, Q. 'Core–shell PLGA/collagen nanofibers loaded with recombinant FN/CDHs as bone tissue engineering scaffolds.' *Connect. Tissue Res.* 55 (2014): 292–298.
77. Liao, I. C.; Chen, S.; Liu, J. B.; Leong, K. W. 'Sustained viral gene delivery through core–shell fibers.' *J. Control. Release* 139 (2009): 48–55.
78. Saraf, A.; Baggett, L. S.; Raphael, R. M.; Kasper, F. K.; Mikos, A. G. 'Regulated non-viral gene delivery from coaxial electrospun fiber mesh scaffolds.' *J. Control. Release* 143 (2010): 95–103.
79. Townsend-Nicholson, A.; Jayasinghe, S. N. 'Cell electrospinning: A unique biotechnique for encapsulating living organisms for generating active biological microthreads/scaffolds.' *Biomacromol.* 7 (2006): 3364–3369.
80. Jayasinghe, S. N.; Irvine, S.; McEwan, J. R. 'Cell electrospinning highly concentrated cellular suspensions containign primary living organisms into cell-bearing threads and scaffolds.' *Nanomed.* 2 (2007): 555–567.
81. Sampson, S. L.; Saraiva, L.; Gustafsson, K.; Jayasinghe, S. N.; Robertson, B. D. 'Cell electrospinning: An *in vitro* and *in vivo* study.' *Small* 10 (2014): 78–82.
82. Ehler, E.; Jayasinghe, S. N. 'Cell electrospinning cardiac patches for tissue engineering the heart.' *Analyst* 139 (2014): 4449–4452.
83. (a) Arumuganathar, S.; Irvine, S.; McEwan, J. R.; Jayasinghe, S. N. 'A novel direct aerodynamically assisted threading methodology for generating biologically viable microthreads encapsulating living primary cells.' *J. Appl. Polym. Sci.* 107 (2008): 1215–1225; (b) Poncelet, D.; de Vos, P.; Suter, N.; Jayasinghe, S. N. 'Bio-electrospraying and cell electrospinning: Progress and opportunities for basic biology and clinical sciences.' *Adv. Healthcare Mater.* 1 (2012): 27–34.
84. Han, D.; Steckl, A. J. 'Superhydrophobic and oleophobic fibers by coaxial electrospinning.' *Langmuir* 25 (2009): 9454–9462.
85. Luo, C. J.; Edirisinghe, M. 'Core-liquid-induced transition from coaxial electrospray to electrospinning of low-viscosity poly(lactide-co-glycolide) sheath solution.' *Macromolecules* 47 (2014): 7930–7938.
86. Yu, D.-G.; Branford-White, C. J.; Chatterton, N. P.; White, K.; Zhu, L.-M.; Shen, X.-X.; Nie, W. 'Electrospinning of concentrated polymer solutions.' *Macromolecules* 43 (2010): 10743–10746.
87. Yu, D. G.; Branford-White, C.; Bligh, S. W.; White, K.; Chatterton, N. P.; Zhu, L. M. 'Improving polymer nanofiber quality using a modified co-axial electrospinning process.' *Macromol. Rapid Commun.* 32 (2011): 744–750.

88. Yu, D. G.; Lu, P.; Branford-White, C.; Yang, J. H.; Wang, X. 'Polyacrylonitrile nanofibers prepared using coaxial electrospinning with LiCl solution as sheath fluid.' *Nanotechnol.* 22 (2011): 435301.
89. Yan, J.; Yu, D.-G. 'Smoothening electrospinning and obtaining high-quality cellulose acetate nanofibers using a modified coaxial process.' *J. Mater. Sci.* 47 (2012): 7138–7147.
90. Wang, X.; Yu, D. G.; Li, X. Y.; Bligh, S. W.; Williams, G. R. 'Electrospun medicated shellac nanofibers for colon-targeted drug delivery.' *Int. J. Pharm.* 490 (2015): 384–390.
91. Yu, D.-G.; Williams, G. R.; Gao, L.-D.; Bligh, S. W. A.; Yang, J.-H.; Wang, X. 'Coaxial electrospinning with sodium dodecylbenzene sulfonate solution for high quality polyacrylonitrile nanofibers.' *Colloids Surf. A* 396 (2012): 161–168.
92. Yu, D. G.; Zhou, J.; Chatterton, N. P.; Li, Y.; Huang, J.; Wang, X. 'Polyacrylonitrile nanofibers coated with silver nanoparticles using a modified coaxial electrospinning process.' *Int. J. Nanomedicine* 7 (2012): 5725–5732.
93. Xie, J.; Mao, H.; Yu, D.-G.; Williams, G. R.; Jin, M. 'Highly stable coated polyvinylpyrrolidone nanofibers prepared using modified coaxial electrospinning.' *Fiber. Polym.* 15 (2014): 78–83.
94. Yu, D. G.; Yu, J. H.; Chen, L.; Williams, G. R.; Wang, X. 'Modified coaxial electrospinning for the preparation of high-quality ketoprofen-loaded cellulose acetate nanofibers.' *Carbohydr. Polym.* 90 (2012): 1016–1023.
95. Huang, W.; Zou, T.; Li, S.; Jing, J.; Xia, X.; Liu, X. 'Drug-loaded zein nanofibers prepared using a modified coaxial electrospinning process.' *AAPS PharmSciTech* 14 (2013): 675–681.
96. Yu, D.-G.; Xu, Y.; Li, Z.; Du, L.-P.; Zhao, B.-G.; Wang, X. 'Coaxial electrospinning with mixed solvents: From flat to round Eudragit L100 nanofibers for better colon-targeted sustained drug release profiles.' *J. Nanomater.* 2014 (2014): 967295.
97. Wu, Y.-H.; Yang, C.; Li, X.-Y.; Zhu, J.-Y.; Yu, D.-G. 'Medicated nanofibers fabricated using NaCl solutions as shell fluids in modified coaxial electrospinning.' *J. Nanomater.* 2016 (2016): 8970213.
98. Yan, J.; White, K.; Yu, D.-G.; Zhao, X.-Y. 'Sustained-release multiple-component cellulose acetate nanofibers fabricated using a modified coaxial electrospinning process.' *J. Mater. Sci.* 49 (2013): 538–547.
99. Qian, W.; Yu, D.-G.; Li, Y.; Li, X.-Y.; Liao, Y.-Z.; Wang, X. 'Triple-component drug-loaded nanocomposites prepared using a modified coaxial electrospinning.' *J. Nanomater.* 2013 (2013): 826471.
100. Yu, D. G.; Zhu, L. M.; Bligh, S. W.; Branford-White, C.; White, K. N. 'Coaxial electrospinning with organic solvent for controlling the size of self-assembled nanoparticles.' *Chem. Commun.* 47 (2011): 1216–1218.
101. Qian, W.; Yu, D. G.; Li, Y.; Liao, Y. Z.; Wang, X.; Wang, L. 'Dual drug release electrospun core–shell nanofibers with tunable dose in the second phase.' *Int. J. Mol. Sci.* 15 (2014): 774–786.

102. Yu, D.-G.; Li, X.-Y.; Wang, X.; Chian, W.; Liao, Y.-Z.; Li, Y. 'Zero-order drug release cellulose acetate nanofibers prepared using coaxial electrospinning.' *Cellulose* 20 (2012): 379–389.
103. Yu, D.-G.; Chian, W.; Wang, X.; Li, X.-Y.; Li, Y.; Liao, Y.-Z. 'Linear drug release membrane prepared by a modified coaxial electrospinning process.' *J. Membrane Sci.* 428 (2013): 150–156.
104. Lallave, M.; Bedia, J.; Ruiz-Rosas, R.; Rodríguez-Mirasol, J.; Cordero, T.; Otero, J. C.; Marquez, M.; Barrero, A.; Loscertales, I. G. 'Filled and hollow carbon nanofibers by coaxial electrospinning of alcell lignin without binder polymers.' *Adv. Mater.* 19 (2007): 4292–4296.
105. Kalra, V.; Lee, J. H.; Park, J. H.; Marquez, M.; Joo, Y. L. 'Confined assembly of asymmetric block-copolymer nanofibers via multiaxial jet electrospinning.' *Small* 5 (2009): 2323–2332.
106. Jiang, S.; Duan, G.; Zussman, E.; Greiner, A.; Agarwal, S. 'Highly flexible and tough concentric triaxial polystyrene fibers.' *ACS Appl. Mater. Interfaces* 6 (2014): 5918–5923.
107. Han, D.; Steckl, A. J. 'Triaxial electrospun nanofiber membranes for controlled dual release of functional molecules.' *ACS Appl. Mater. Interfaces* 5 (2013): 8241–8245.
108. Yu, D. G.; Li, X. Y.; Wang, X.; Yang, J. H.; Bligh, S. W.; Williams, G. R. 'Nanofibers fabricated using triaxial electrospinning as zero order drug delivery systems.' *ACS Appl. Mater. Interfaces* 7 (2015): 18891–18897.
109. Yang, C.; Yu, D. G.; Pan, D.; Liu, X. K.; Wang, X.; Bligh, S. W.; Williams, G. R. 'Electrospun pH-sensitive core–shell polymer nanocomposites fabricated using a tri-axial process.' *Acta Biomater.* 35 (2016): 77–86.
110. Yang, G. Z.; Li, J. J.; Yu, D. G.; He, M. F.; Yang, J. H.; Williams, G. R. 'Nanosized sustained-release drug depots fabricated using modified tri-axial electrospinning.' *Acta Biomater.* 53 (2017): 233–241.
111. Khalf, A.; Singarapu, K.; Madihally, S. V. 'Influence of solvent characteristics in triaxial electrospun fiber formation.' *Reactive Funct. Polym.* 90 (2015): 36–46.
112. Labbaf, S.; Ghanbar, H.; Stride, E.; Edirisinghe, M. 'Preparation of multilayered polymeric structures using a novel four-needle coaxial electrohydrodynamic device.' *Macromol. Rapid Commun.* 35 (2014): 618–623.

5

A Comprehensive Study of Side-by-Side Electrospinning

5.1 Introduction

Side-by-side electrospinning is a two-liquid process, and in many ways can be regarded as a companion technique to coaxial spinning. Rather than the two liquids being nested inside one another as in the coaxial process, however, they are placed adjacent to one another (Figure 5.1(a)). As for coaxial spinning, the structure of the spinneret is propagated into the solid products, and this should result in so-called Janus fibres with the two sides different (Figure 5.1(b)).

Janus fibres differ from core/shell fibres in that both parts of the fibre are in contact with the surrounding milieu, while in a core/shell fibre the shell protects the core. Thus, while for core/shell fibres drug release from the shell will occur prior to release from the core, release from the two sides of the Janus fibres can occur concomitantly. This is potentially very useful. For instance, fibres with the two sides made from different polymers could be prepared with a different drug loaded in each, to release the two individual active ingredients at the same time but with different rates. This delivery modality might also be delivered with a mixture of two different types of monolithic fibre, but with such a mixture there is a risk of the two fibre populations separating during the release process. This might result in the two drugs being released in different parts of the body. With the Janus materials, each individual fibre has two sides and contains both drugs, so even if the fibre mat breaks up the two drugs will still be delivered concomitantly.

The first report of side-by-side spinning came from Gupta and Wilkes in 2003.[1] These authors prepared fibres where one side comprised

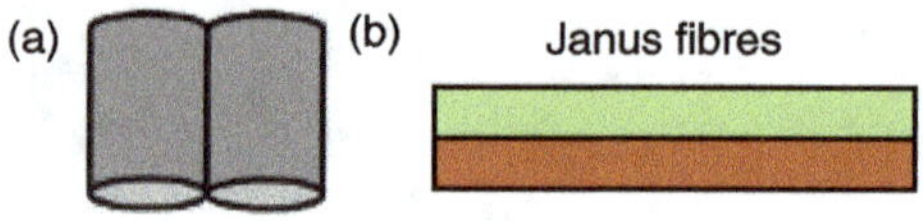

Figure 5.1 The use of side-by-side electrospinning to prepare Janus fibres. (a) The side-by-side spinneret, and (b) the resultant Janus fibres.

poly(vinyl chloride) (PVC) and polyurethane (PU), and the other PVC/poly(vinylidene fluoride) (PVDF). Since then there have been a few more reports of Janus fibres, but despite its great potential this area of work has received much less attention than coaxial electrospinning.

5.2 Experimental considerations

5.2.1 Challenges in side-by-side spinning

The main reason for the paucity of reports of Janus fibres from side-by-side electrospinning arises from the difficulty in generating integrated and homogeneous products when a standard spinneret is used. In the coaxial (or indeed triaxial) modality, the liquids are nested one inside another, and the charge imparted at the spinneret is spread across the liquid jet as it is emitted. This means that the liquids travel together from the Taylor cone towards the collector, and in general core/shell-type architectures are obtained. However, with the side-by-side spinneret the two liquids emerge from adjacent needles, with both bearing the same charge polarity and only a small interfacial contact area. This will lead to extensive Coulombic repulsions between the two jets at the Taylor cone and beyond, and tends to cause separation of the two liquids.

The properties of the two liquids being processed also need to be carefully considered: for successful production of a Janus fibre, it is important for them to behave in a similar fashion under the influence of the electrical field. If one liquid charges or dries much faster than the other, this is likely to lead to phase separation and clogging of the needle.

Because of this difficulty, the majority of electrospun Janus fibres prepared to date use the same polymer for both working liquids. For instance, Liu's group have prepared Janus fibres with magnetic–fluorescent properties using poly(methyl methacrylate) for both sides.[2] In other work, Lv *et al.* have generated Janus CeO_2/SiO_2 fibres by first spinning two poly(vinyl pyrrolidone) (PVP) solutions containing inorganic precursors and then calcining the product.[3] Liu and co-workers

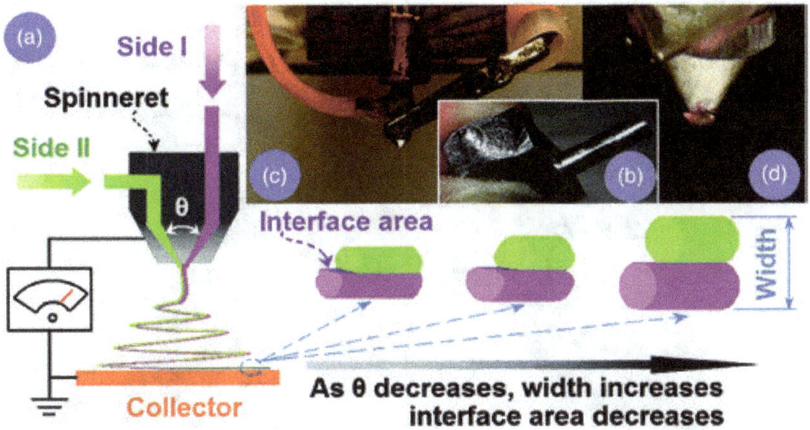

Figure 5.2 Varying the angle between the capillaries in a side-by-side electrospinning experiment, showing (a) the spinneret design with the angle θ marked; (b) a photograph of the spinneret; (c) the experimental set-up; and (d) the compound Taylor cone. (Reproduced with permission from Chen, G.; Xu, Y.; Yu, D. G.; Zhang, D. F.; Chatterton, N. P.; White, K. N. 'Structure-tunable Janus fibers fabricated using spinnerets with varying port angles.' *Chem. Commun.* 51 (2015): 4623–4626. Copyright Royal Society of Chemistry 2015.)

have similarly used Janus fibres with both sides based on PVP as sacrificial templates to yield inorganic materials.[4]

5.2.2 Spinneret design

The simplest design one can envisage for side-by-side spinning comprises two metal capillaries aligned in a parallel manner, as shown in Figure 5.1(a). Although there are a number of issues with this, as identified above, some researchers have successfully used such a spinneret to generate Janus products.[4, 5] It has been shown by Chen *et al.* that the angle between the two capillaries can be varied to adjust the width of the two sides of the Janus fibres produced.[6] In this work, solutions of Eudragit L100 and PVP were electrospun through a side-by-side spinneret with the angle between the two capillaries varied between 40 and 70° (Figure 5.2). An increasing angle led to narrower fibres, and the central interface between the two sides of the fibre became less distinct (Figure 5.3). The flow rates of the two sides could also be varied to tune the composition of the electrospun products. In this specific case, the

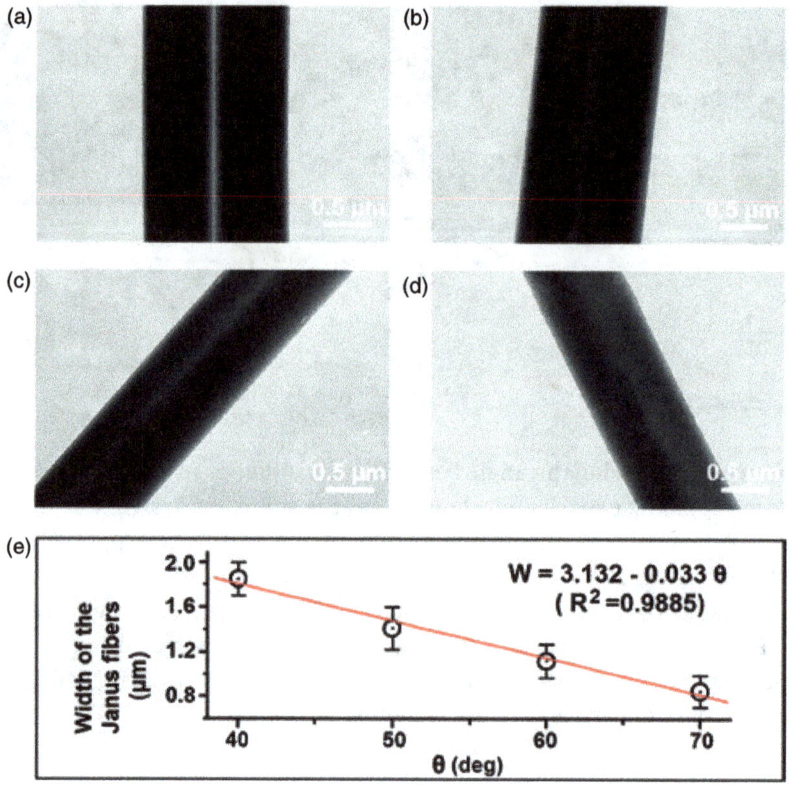

Figure 5.3 Fibres produced with angles of (a) 40; (b) 50; (c) 60; and (d) 70° between the spinneret ports. (e) The relationship between the fibre diameter and angle. (Reproduced with permission from Chen, G.; Xu, Y.; Yu, D. G.; Zhang, D. F.; Chatterton, N. P.; White, K. N. 'Structure-tunable Janus fibers fabricated using spinnerets with varying port angles.' *Chem. Commun.* 51 (2015): 4623–4626. Copyright Royal Society of Chemistry 2015.)

PVP side of the fibres was loaded with rhodamine B (a pink dye) and the Eudragit side with 8-anilino-1-naphthalenesulfonic acid ammonium salt (a fluorescent probe), and altering the flow rates of the two sides allowed the colour of the fibres under ultraviolet light to be varied.

To overcome the issues identified above using a spinneret simply comprising two parallel needles, a number of different approaches have been explored. These focus on preventing the two liquids from separating when they leave the spinneret. One approach, used by Ma *et al.*, is to feed the liquids into a plastic nozzle after they exit the parallel metal

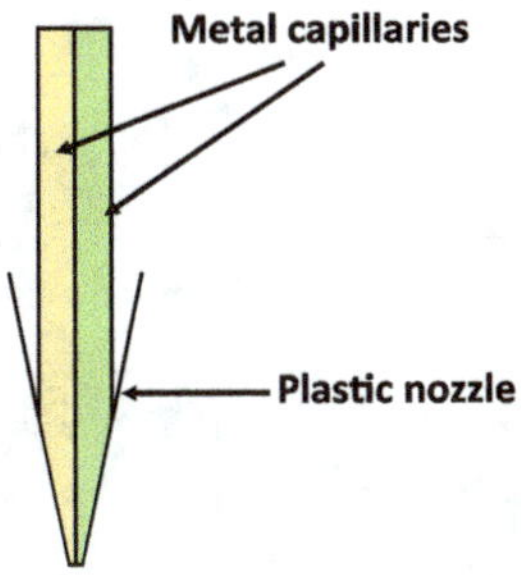

Figure 5.4 The spinneret developed by Ma *et al.*[7]

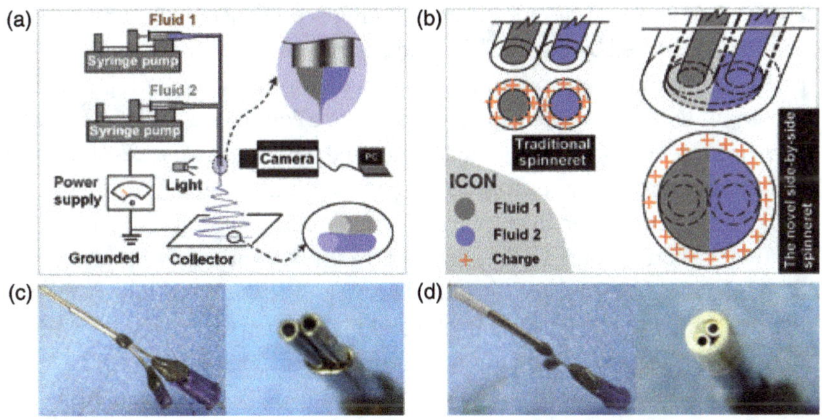

Figure 5.5 A Teflon-coated side-by-side spinneret. Schematics are shown of (a) the experimental set-up and (b) the charge localisation around the spinnerets during electrospinning. Pictures of the (c) side-by-side and (d) Teflon-coated spinneret are also shown. (Reproduced with permission from Yu, D. G.; Yang, C.; Jin, M.; Williams, G. R.; Zou, H.; Wang, X.; Annie Bligh, S. W. 'Medicated Janus fibers fabricated using a Teflon-coated side-by-side spinneret.' *Colloids Surf. B* 138 (2016): 110–116. Copyright Elsevier 2016.)

capillaries.[7] This is depicted schematically in Figure 5.4. The nozzle holds the two liquids together as they exit the spinneret, increasing the contact area between them, spreading the charge around the exterior of the two liquids and helping to ensure homogeneous Janus products.

Yu *et al.* have employed a similar spinneret design, using a short length of Teflon tube to coat the parallel capillaries (Figure 5.5).[8] The coating performs the same role as the plastic nozzle used by Ma. It was

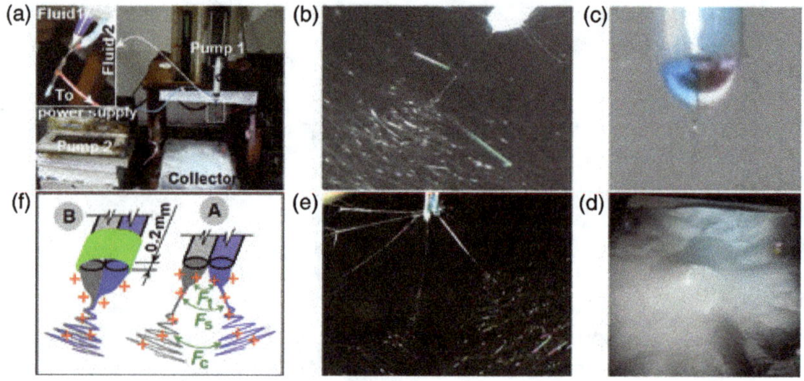

Figure 5.6 The side-by-side electrospinning process using a Teflon coated spinneret explored by Yu *et al.*[8] (a) The experimental set-up; (b) a digital photgraph of the electrospinning process with the Teflon-coated spinneret; (c) use of the Teflon-coated spinneret leads to a compound Taylor cone with two distinct sides; (d) the fibre mat generated with the uncoated spinneret is clearly inhomogeneous, as a result of the two solutions separating on exiting the spinneret, as shown in (e); (f) a schematic of the influence of the Teflon coating: (A) an uncoated spinneret leads to the separation of the working liquids because of repulsive forces F_t (between the two Taylor cones), F_s (between the two straight liquid jets) and F_c (between the two coils), while in (B) the Teflon coating encourages formation of an integrated Janus Taylor cone. (Reproduced with permission from Yu, D. G.; Yang, C.; Jin, M.; Williams, G. R.; Zou, H.; Wang, X.; Annie Bligh, S. W. 'Medicated Janus fibers fabricated using a Teflon-coated side-by-side spinneret.' *Colloids Surf. B* 138 (2016): 110–116. Copyright Elsevier 2016.)

found that a smooth and continuous spinning process could be performed using the Teflon coating, leading to homogeneous fibres with clear Janus structure. The use of a dye in each of the liquids allowed the authors to see a clear compound Taylor cone (Figure 5.6). However, when the experiment was undertaken without the coating, the two liquids were observed to separate upon exiting the spinneret, resulting in a fibre mat which was visibly inhomogeneous (Figure 5.6). The addition of the Teflon coating is thus crucial for a successful experimental set-up. A microfluidic device has been employed as the spinneret to similar ends by Lin *et al.*[9] In this approach, the two liquids flow adjacent to one another and in contact for some time before exiting the device.

An alternative route to ensure high-quality Janus structures was reported in some recent work.[10] Rather than placing the two capillaries

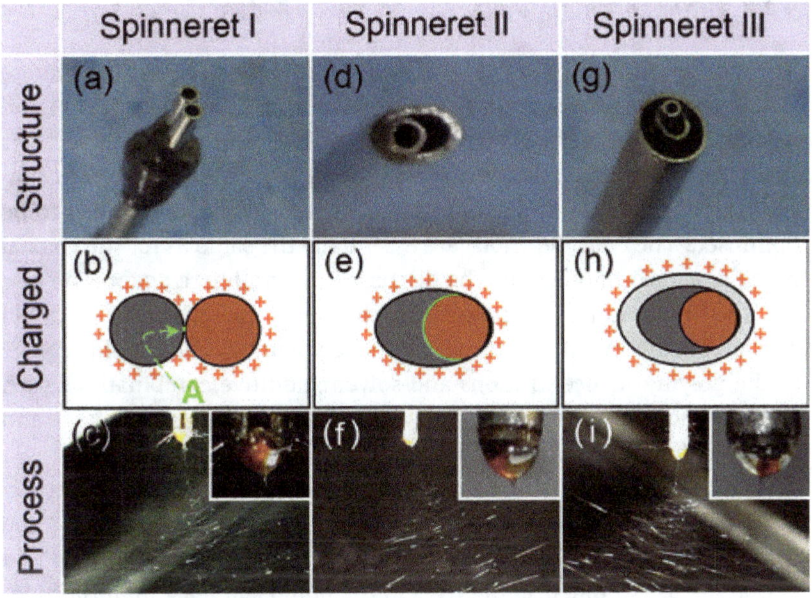

Figure 5.7 Different spinnerets explored for side-by-side electrospinning by Yu *et al.*[10] The standard side-by-side spinneret is shown in (a); this leads to a small contact area between the two liquids (b), and as a result (c) the polymer solutions tend to separate when leaving the spinneret. Using a nested 'acentric' spinneret (d) spreads the charge around the exterior of the two liquids (e), leading to much less separation, as depicted in (f). The addition of a shell compartment (g) improves the situation still further, (h) spreading the charge over the shell compartment and (i) resulting in smooth electrospinning processes with no separation of the two polymer components. (Reproduced with permission from Yu, D. G.; Li, J. J.; Zhang, M.; Williams, G. R. 'High quality Janus nanofibers prepared using three-fluid electrospinning,' *Chem. Commun*. 53 (2017): 4542–4545. Copyright Royal Society of Chemistry 2017.)

of the spinneret adjacent to one another, Yu *et al.* took a different approach of nesting one capillary inside another (a so-called 'acentric spinneret'; Figure 5.7). When working with PVP and shellac solutions, this led to a reduced tendency for the two polymer solutions to separate upon leaving the spinneret and the observation of more integrated Janus structures. The quality of the fibres produced was improved again if the acentric spinneret was incorporated in the centre of a larger needle and a pure solvent flowed around the outside of the two polymer solutions.

5.2.3 Other considerations

In order to establish a successful electrospinning process to generate Janus fibres, in addition to the spinneret design the same solution and processing parameters as have been discussed previously (see sections 2.5, 3.2 and 4.2) must be considered. The voltage, solvent, polymer concentration, flow rate and spinneret-to-collector distance all need to be optimised. The considerations are essentially the same as for the coaxial process, and so they will not be discussed in detail here again. The rate at which the two liquids charge and dry under the electrical field will be particularly important for side-by-side spinning, and careful choice of the polymer concentrations and solvent/additive combinations such that both liquids can be successfully processed with the same voltage and spinneret-to-collector distance will be required.

As for the coaxial experiment, we recommend that the starting point for a side-by-side process is to understand and optimise the spinning of the two liquids individually before moving on to two-liquid work. The use of one or more dyes in the liquids, at least in initial side-by-side experiments, can be very beneficial to visualise the Taylor cone to ensure there are two clear compartments with no blending of the liquids.

5.3 Janus fibres in drug delivery

At the time of writing, there are only three reports of the use of Janus fibres in drug delivery. The first comes from Yu and co-workers, who used a Teflon-coated spinneret to facilitate the production of high-quality Janus fibres.[8] One side of the fibres was made of PVP, and the other of ethyl cellulose (EC) with small amounts of PVP doped in it. Ketoprofen (KET) was used as a model drug, and incorporated into both sides of the fibres. The intention was to produce biphasic drug delivery systems, with the PVP compartment dissolving rapidly to release a loading dose of KET and rapidly raise the plasma concentration into the therapeutic window. The EC side then provides extended drug release, ensuring a therapeutic concentration of the drug is maintained for a sustained period of time. Clear Janus structures were produced, as shown in Figure 5.8(a). Varying the amount of PVP doped into the EC side of the fibres permitted the second (sustained) phase of release to be tuned, with greater PVP contents resulting in both more rapid release and also in a larger overall release percentage (Figure 5.8(b)).

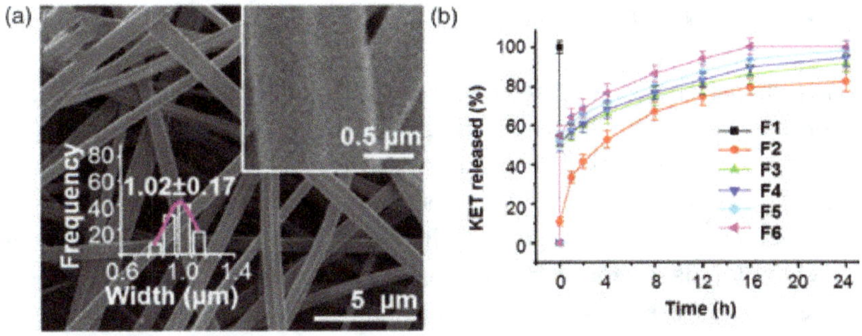

Figure 5.8 Biphasic release from electrospun Janus fibres. (a) Fibres prepared with one side comprising poly(vinyl pyrrolidone) (PVP)/ ketoprofen (KET) and the other ethyl cellulose (EC)/KET doped with a small amount of PVP; (b) the effect of changing the PVP content in the EC side of the fibres on the release profile. F1 and F2 are control fibres made of PVP/KET and EC/KET, respectively, and F3–F6 are Janus fibres with increasing amounts of PVP in the EC side (F3: 0% w/w PVP; F4: 3.7%; F5: 7.1%; F6: 16.1%). The pure PVP fibres (F1) lead to very rapid release, while the pure EC fibres (F2) free the drug into solution only very slowly. The Janus fibres combine both these release modalities, to provide an initial burst of release followed by sustained release. Increasing amounts of PVP in the EC side of the fibres lead both to more rapid release in the sustained phase, and also to a greater extent of release being reached overall. (Reproduced with permission from Yu, D. G.; Yang, C.; Jin, M.; Williams, G. R.; Zou, H.; Wang, X.; Annie Bligh, S. W. 'Medicated Janus fibers fabricated using a Teflon-coated side-by-side spinneret.' *Colloids Surf. B* 138 (2016): 110–116. Copyright Elsevier 2016.)

Similar biphasic release has been reported for fibres prepared using poly(acrylonitrile) (PAN) and PVP for the two sides.[11] Most recently, Yu's team used an acentric spinneret (see section 5.2.2) to prepare Janus fibres with both sides comprising PVP.[12] One spinning solution was made from a high-molecular-weight and electrospinnable PVP (molecular weight (Mw) = 360 kDa) and contained helicid as a model drug. The second comprised an unspinnable solution of PVP (Mw = 8 kDa) and sodium dodecyl sulfate (SDS; a permeation enhancer). It proved possible to generate Janus fibres from these two solutions, showing that, just as with coaxial electrospinning, only one fluid need be individually electrospinnable to yield fibres. The fibres led to rapid release of helicid, and the presence of SDS accelerated the permeation of the drug through porcine sublingual mucosae *ex vivo*.

5.4 Conclusions

This chapter has considered the possibility of preparing Janus fibres from side-by-side electrospinning. These structures are companion structures to the core/shell architecture resulting from coaxial spinning. The side-by-side experiment is much more technically challenging to implement than coaxial spinning, however, because of the tendency of the two liquids to separate upon exiting the spinneret. As a result, there is very little work reporting Janus fibres for drug delivery. However, the results reported to date do suggest that they have potential in this field. Encouragingly, a number of significant improvements to the experimental protocol have recently been developed, leading to much higher-quality Janus products being generated. It is expected that these will permit researchers to accelerate progress in this field over the coming years, such that the true potential of Janus nanofibres in drug delivery can be realised.

5.5 References

1. Gupta, P.; Wilkes, G. L. 'Some investigations on the fiber formation by utilizing a side-by-side bicomponent electrospinning approach.' *Polymer* 44 (2003): 6353–6359.
2. Ma, Q.; Yu, W.; Dong, X.; Wang, J.; Liu, G. 'Janus nanobelts: Fabrication, structure and enhanced magnetic-fluorescent bifunctional performance.' *Nanoscale* 6 (2014): 2945–2952; Tian, J.; Ma, Q.; Dong, X.; Yu, W.; Yang, M.; Yang, Y.; Wang, J.; Liu, G. 'Flexible Janus nanoribbons to help obtain simultaneous color-tunable enhanced photoluminescence, magnetism and electrical conduction trifunctionality.' *RSC Adv.* 6 (2016): 36180–36191.
3. Lv, N.; Wang, Z.; Bi, W.; Li, G.; Zhang, J.; Ni, J. 'C8-modified CeO_2/SiO_2 Janus fibers for selective capture and individual MS detection of low-abundance peptides and phosphopeptides.' *J. Mater. Chem. B* 4 (2016): 4402–4409.
4. Liu, Z.; Sun, D. D.; Guo, P.; Leckie, J. O. 'An efficient bicomponent TiO_2/SnO_2 nanofiber photocatalyst fabricated by electrospinning with a side-by-side dual spinneret method.' *Nano Lett.* 7 (2007): 1081–1085.
5. Starr, J. D.; Andrew, J. S. 'Janus-type bi-phasic functional nanofibers.' *Chem. Commun.* 49 (2013): 4151–4153; Chen, S.; Hou, H.; Hu, P.; Wendorff, J. H.; Greiner, A.; Agarwal, S. 'Effect of different bicomponent electrospinning techniques on the formation of polymeric nanosprings.' *Macromol. Mater. Eng.* 294 (2009): 781–786.

6. Chen, G.; Xu, Y.; Yu, D. G.; Zhang, D. F.; Chatterton, N. P.; White, K. N. 'Structure-tunable Janus fibers fabricated using spinnerets with varying port angles.' *Chem. Commun.* 51 (2015): 4623–4626.
7. Ma, Q.; Wang, J.; Dong, X.; Yu, W.; Liu, G. 'Flexible Janus nanoribbons array: A new strategy to achieve excellent electrically conductive anisotropy, magnetism, and photoluminescence.' *Adv. Funct. Mater* 25 (2015): 2436–2443.
8. Yu, D. G.; Yang, C.; Jin, M.; Williams, G. R.; Zou, H.; Wang, X.; Annie Bligh, S. W. 'Medicated Janus fibers fabricated using a Teflon-coated side-by-side spinneret.' *Colloids Surf. B* 138 (2016): 110–116.
9. Lin, T.; Wang, H.; Wang, X. 'Self-crimping bicomponent nanofibers electrospun from polyacrylonitrile and elastomeric polyurethane.' *Adv. Mater.* 17 (2005): 2699–2703.
10. Yu, D. G.; Li, J. J.; Zhang, M.; Williams, G. R. 'High-quality Janus nanofibers prepared using three-fluid electrospinning.' *Chem. Commun.* 53 (2017): 4542–4545.
11. Geng, Y.; Zhang, P.; Wang, Q.; Liu, Y.; Pan, K. 'Novel PAN/PVP Janus ultrafine fiber membrane and its application for biphasic drug release.' *J. Mater. Chem. B* 5 (2017): 5390–5396.
12. Wang, K.; Liu, X.-K.; Chen, X.-H.; Yu, D.-G.; Yang, Y.-Y.; Liu, P. 'Electrospun hydrophilic Janus nanocomposites for the rapid onset of therapeutic action of helicid.' *ACS Appl. Mater. Interfaces* 10 (2018): 2859–2867.

6

Nanofibre Fabrication: Alternative Approaches

6.1 Introduction

The previous chapters have all focused on electrospinning as the means of fibre formation, since this is the technique which has to date received by far the most research attention. There exists a range of other, less explored, technologies for fibre production, however, and these will all be discussed briefly in the context of drug delivery in this chapter. Further details on the principles of many of these techniques can be found in recent reviews by Luo *et al.*[1] and Qi and Craig.[2]

6.2 Alternating current electrospinning

Electricity comprises a flow of electrons (negatively charged subatomic particles). In direct current (DC; used for the vast majority of electrospinning work) the electrons flow in one direction continually. It is also possible to have alternating current (AC), which is used to power most electrical devices in the home. AC involves a periodic change in the direction of current flow: that is, the electrons first flow in one direction and then switch to flow in the reverse direction. The switch between directions is repeated many times per second and is known as the frequency of the AC. Using an AC power supply rather than the conventional DC supply was first shown to generate polymer-based nanofibres in 2004.[3]

The experimental set-up for AC electrospinning is similar to that for the DC process, but it does not require a grounded collector. Because

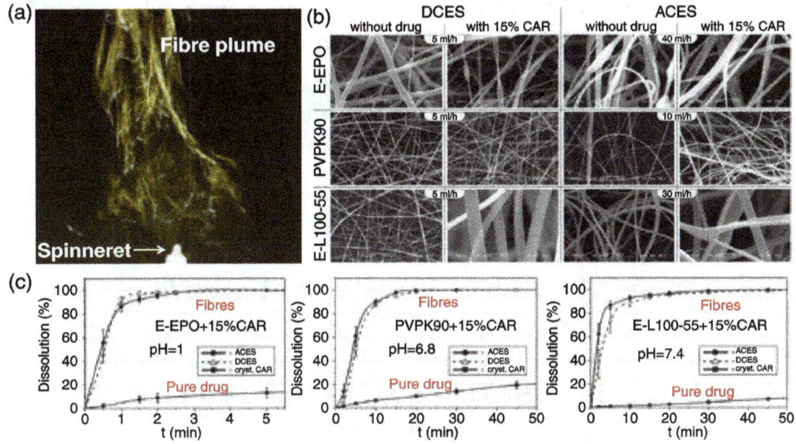

Figure 6.1 Alternating current electrospinning for fibre production. (a) The plume of fibres produced; (b) fibres produced from direct current electrospinning (DCES) and alternating current electrospinning (ACES) (E: Eudragit; CAR: carvedilol); (c) dissolution profiles for the fibres. (Adapted with permission from Balogh, A.; Cselko, R.; Demuth, B.; Verreck, G.; Mensch, J.; Marosi, G.; Nagy, Z. K. 'Alternating current electrospinning for preparation of fibrous drug delivery systems.' *Int. J. Pharm.* 495 (2015): 75–80. Copyright Elsevier 2015.)

the current alternates, the fibres produced at one instant in time carry a positive charge, while those generated shortly thereafter have a negative charge. The positive and negative fibres thus discharge on each other, which results in an aerogel plume of fibres, as depicted in Figure 6.1(a). The frequency of the AC current determines whether charge carriers of one polarity have sufficient time to charge the solution and result in spinning. The optimal AC frequency is material-dependent and typically in the range of 50 Hz–1 kHz.[4]

The AC approach has been explored for the fabrication of drug-loaded fibres in a few recent studies. In one, Balogh *et al.* undertook a direct comparison of fibres prepared by DC and AC spinning.[5] They used the beta-blocker carvedilol as a model drug, and fibres were generated using three different polymers: Eudragit EPO, a cationic copolymer soluble below pH 5.0; Eudragit L100-55, an anionic polymer soluble above pH 5.5; and the neutral polymer poly(vinyl pyrrolidone) (PVP). It was found that fibres could be generated with all three polymers from both types of spinning (Figure 6.1(b)), but that it was possible to use much faster flow rates in the AC process. With DC spinning, a maximum flow rate of 5 ml h^{-1} could be achieved, whereas with AC this could be increased to up to 40 ml h^{-1}. All fibres, from both processes and made from all polymers, existed as amorphous solid dispersions. The drug release profiles were studied, and the AC and DC fibres were found to be indistinguishable in their performance (Figure 6.1(c)).

The same team have also compared AC and DC electrospinning of blends of hydroxypropylmethylcellulose (HPMC) and poly(ethylene oxide) (PEO) with the poorly water-soluble diuretic spironolactone.[6] Both HPMC and PEO alone could be processed by the DC approach. In contrast, AC electrospinning of HPMC led to a mixture of droplets and fibres, and high-molecular-weight PEOs did not yield any solid products at all in the AC method. Selecting appropriate blends of the two polymers, however, permitted high-quality fibres to be formed via AC spinning.

AC processing of HPMC or PEO with spironolactone also proved to be problematic, but again with the right mix of HPMC and PEO drug-loaded fibres could be generated. These were able to accelerate the dissolution rate of the drug, even at loadings of up to 40% w/w. The AC-generated fibres were found to be several orders of magnitude thinner than the DC electrospun fibres despite the flow rate being three times faster in the AC process.

Similar observations have been reported using HPMC acetate succinate (HPMCAS) and spironolactone.[7] HPMCAS could not be processed by either DC or AC electrospinning; the addition of PEO permitted fibres to be produced with the DC approach, but not using AC, and the addition of an ionic surfactant or salt was required to produce high-quality fibres with AC spinning. As with HPMC, the HPMCAS fibres led to a significant enhancement in the dissolution rate.

It is thus clear that AC electrospinning is similarly effective to the DC approach in producing drug delivery systems. Although its use in this regard is in its infancy, given the fact it allows higher throughput than the DC technique, it seems certain that this is an approach which is likely to receive much more attention in the coming years.

6.3 Melt electrospinning

Another variant of electrospinning which has attracted some attention in the drug delivery sphere is the melt process. This is discussed in detail in a recent review.[8] In brief, the process is analogous to the solution electrospinning discussed in previous chapters, but in place of a

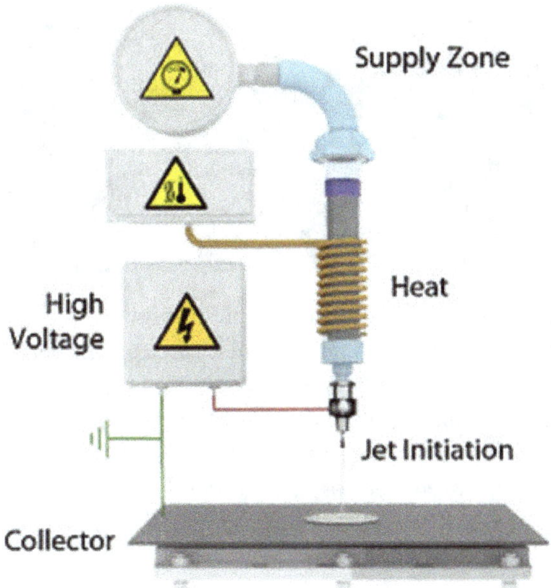

Figure 6.2 The apparatus used for melt electrospinning. (Reproduced with permission from Brown, T. D.; Dalton, P. D.; Hutmacher, D. W. 'Melt electrospinning today: An opportune time for an emerging polymer process.' *Prog. Polym. Sci.* 56 (2016): 116–166. Copyright Elsevier 2016.)

polymer solution a melt is used. This adds some complexity to the process, because the syringe and spinneret must be heated to maintain the polymer in its liquid state. Further, the elevated temperature can potentially lead to drug degradation, since many drugs are thermally labile. The fibres produced in melt spinning are typically found to have larger diameters than those from the solution route due to the significantly higher viscosity of a polymer melt than its solution form. The apparatus used is depicted in Figure 6.2.

Despite these apparent disadvantages, there are a number of attractive aspects of the melt spinning process, not least the fact that it obviates the need to handle large volumes of volatile solvents. This both renders the process safer, particularly if it is to be performed on the larger scale, and precludes any solvent contamination in the products.

The first report of a melt electrospun drug delivery system came from Nagy and co-workers, who prepared melt-spun fibres of Eudragit

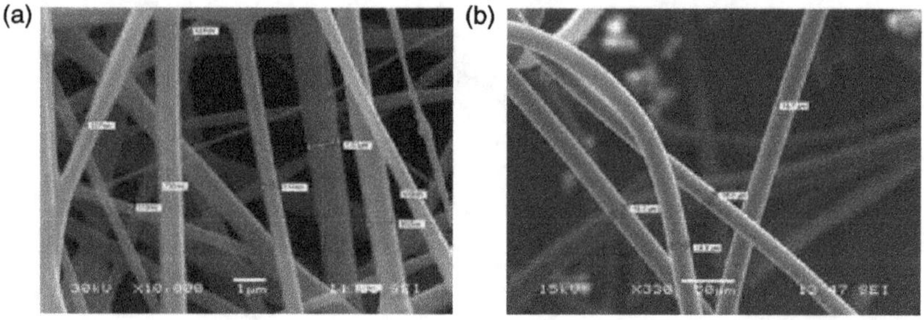

Figure 6.3 Scanning electron microscopy images of Eudragit E / carvedilol fibres prepared by (a) solution and (b) melt electrospinning. (Reproduced with permission from Nagy, Z. K.; Balogh, A.; Dravavolgyi, G.; Ferguson, J.; Pataki, H.; Vajna, B.; Marosi, G. 'Solvent-free melt electrospinning for preparation of fast dissolving drug delivery system and comparison with solvent-based electrospun and melt extruded systems.' *J. Pharm. Sci.* 102 (2013): 508–517. Copyright Elsevier 2013.)

EPO loaded with carvedilol.[9] The drug and polymer were melted and mixed to form a homogeneous solid mixture prior to spinning, and then processed as in a solution experiment but with both the syringe and spinneret heated. The melt fibres were much wider than analogous systems processed through solution spinning, with those from melt processing having diameters of 5–30 μm, as compared to 300–1000 nm for the solution-spun fibres (Figure 6.3). The drug was completely amorphously dispersed in the fibres regardless of the processing route. This is as expected for solution spinning, and in the melt case was thought to be because the experiment was carried out above the melting point of carvedilol. The melt fibres freed their drug loading faster than the solution-spun analogues, despite the much larger surface area of the latter. The authors ascribed this to the fact that the melt fibres had a loose non-woven structure, whereas those prepared by solution spinning were more tightly packed (Figure 6.3).

This work has been built on to blend plasticisers with the polymer Eudragit E and carvedilol active ingredient.[10] The plasticisers triacetin, Tween 80 and polyethylene glycol were all investigated with the goal of reducing the melting point of the polymer/drug blend and thereby permitting lower temperatures to be used for spinning. This should reduce the likelihood of any degradation occurring. High-performance liquid chromatography data obtained on dissolved fibres revealed that the addition of plasticisers clearly reduced the amounts of carvedilol degradation products present after melt spinning.

A direct comparison of poly(ε-caprolactone) (PCL) fibres generated by the melt and solution-spinning approaches has been reported by Lian and Meng.[11] These authors prepared curcumin-loaded fibres of around 4 μm in diameter using both techniques. They found that there was a greater tendency for the curcumin to crystallise using the solution route (a result of its low solubility in the solvent used for spinning). The melt fibres led to a reduced burst release and a slower release rate. These findings were attributed to the solution-spun fibres having a porous structure, which permitted both water ingress and the incorporated curcumin to diffuse out of the polymer matrix.

Melt electrospinning typically generates micron-size fibres. In a recent effort, however, highly uniform and precise deposition of PCL nanofibres (817 ± 165 nm) was achieved using a method known as *melt electrospinning writing*.[12] This combines melt electrospinning with additive manufacturing (three-dimensional (3D) printing) technology, using a computer-controlled extruder moving on a translational stage to build a 3D structure layer by layer. The 3D fibrous architecture produced allowed efficient *in vitro* proliferation of primary human mesenchymal stromal cells. The melt electrospinning writing technology can produce regular 3D morphologies in a highly controllable and reproducible fashion, and is currently being explored for a range of tissue-engineering applications.

Although melt electrospinning has received much less research interest than the solution process, it appears to be equally as flexible in terms of handling multiple fluids, and coaxial melt spinning has been reported.[13] The initial melt spinning experiment is perhaps harder to establish than the solution route, but it is clear that this approach has a great deal of unexplored potential in the development of drug delivery systems.

6.4 Centrifugal spinning

Centrifugal spinning employs a rotating polymer source to generate fibres. Several centrifugal methods can generate nanofibres. These include Forcespinning, which employs rotary speed of above 2000 revolutions per minute (rpm),[14] electrocentrifugal spinning,[15] which combines a strong electric potential (as in electrospinning) with centrifugal force, and pressurised gyration, which adds high pressure (> 10 kPa) to centrifugal spinning to enhance fibre formation (see section 6.8).[16]

These approaches can be applied to polymer solutions and emulsions, and if the source can be heated also to a polymer melt

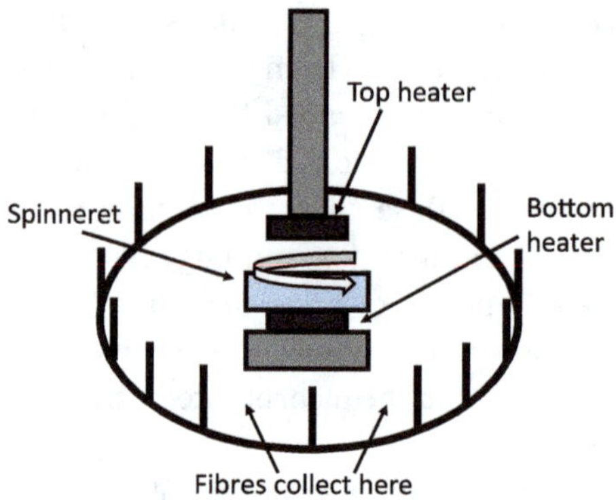

Figure 6.4 A schematic diagram of the apparatus used for centrifugal spinning. (Adapted from Zander, N. E. 'Formation of melt and solution spun polycaprolactone fibers by centrifugal spinning.' *J. Appl. Polym. Sci.* 132 (2015): 41269[18].)

(Figure 6.4).[17] This technique has received some attention in the context of drug delivery. For instance, Zander prepared PCL fibres using both the solution and melt variants of the centrifugal technique.[18] This author employed spinning speeds in the range of 3000–18,000 rpm, yielding fibres of *ca.* 10 μm in diameter. PC12 neuron cells could be successfully grown on the fibres, demonstrating that they have potential in nerve tissue engineering.

In other work, centrifugally spun PCL/PVP fibres containing the antibiotic tetracycline have been produced from a methanol/chloroform solution at 2000 rpm.[19] These were sub-micron in their diameters, and highly aligned. The rate of drug release could be tuned by varying the PCL/PVP ratio in the fibres, and the fibres were found to be effective in inhibiting bacterial growth. Core/shell fibres for the delivery of growth factors have further been reported from centrifugal spinning of a water-in-oil emulsion, with PCL dissolved in the oil phase.[20]

Fibres have also been made using a melt process with sucrose (a sugar dimer) loaded with a range of poorly water-soluble drugs, including olanzapine (an antipsychotic medicine) and piroxicam (a non-steroidal anti-inflammatory).[21] The fibres were 10–15 μm in diameter, and the dissolution rate of the drugs enhanced after fibre formation.

Since the centrifugal spinning approach is a simple one which allows relatively large-scale production of fibres,[22] it appears to have much promise in the drug delivery field. It can also be coupled to electrospinning, with both centrifugal and electrical forces applied simultaneously to drive solvent evaporation.[15] Such centrifugal electrospinning uses the same equipment as the standard centrifugal process but additionally applies a high voltage between the rotating spinneret and the collector. It has been reported to lead to significantly higher throughput than standard electrospinning,[23] and to produce highly aligned fibres.[23b, 24] Centrifugal electrospinning has further been demonstrated to have potential in the production of drug delivery systems, with a recent report of PVP fibres loaded with the antibiotic tetracycline hydrochloride.[25] Production rates of up to 120 g h^{-1} could be realised.

6.5 Solution blowing and melt blowing

A pressurised gas can be exploited to produce nanoscale fibres, starting either with a polymer solution in a technique known as solution blowing or from a molten polymer source (melt blowing). The experimental apparatus used is similar to electrospinning, in that a polymer solution (or melt) is expelled through a needle (spinneret) at a controlled rate. The spinneret is surrounded by an outer nozzle which applies pressured gas to the fluid being expelled, as illustrated in Figure 6.5.[26]

A few studies have explored solution blowing in drug delivery, with the first such work being from Oliveira *et al.* in 2013.[27] These authors prepared poly(lactic acid) (PLA) fibres loaded with the hormone progesterone, which can be used to regulate the reproductive cycle in livestock. Fibres were produced from solutions with 6% w/v PLA and between 0 and 8% w/v progesterone (Figure 6.6(a)). The PLA is semi-crystalline both before and after processing, while the drug is amorphous post-spinning. The fibres behave very similarly in terms of their release behaviour, regardless of the amount of drug loaded (Figure 6.6(b)).

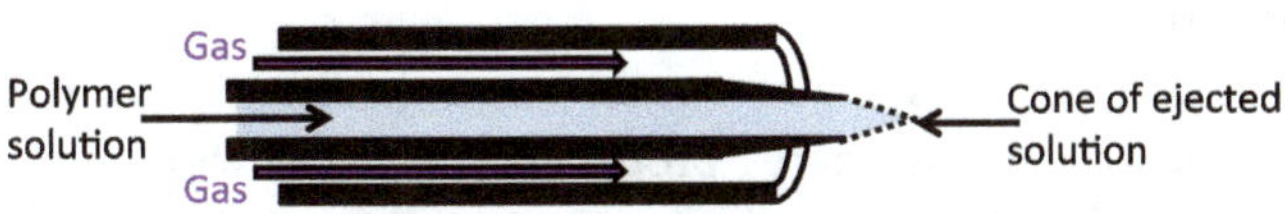

Figure 6.5 The apparatus used for solution blow spinning or melt blowing. (Adapted from Souza, M. A.; Sakamoto, K. Y.; Mattoso, L. H. C. 'Release of the diclofenac sodium by nanofibers of poly(3-hydroxybutyrate-co-3-hydroxyvalerate) obtained from electrospinning and solution blow spinning.' *J. Nanomater.* 2014 (2014): 129035.)

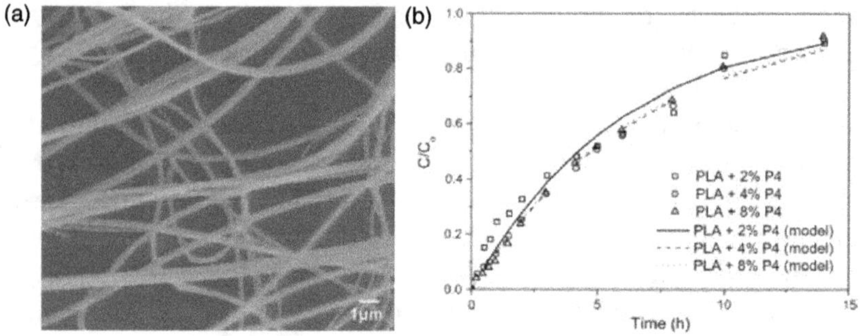

Figure 6.6 Progesterone-loaded poly(lactic acid) (PLA) fibres prepared by solution blowing. (a) A scanning electron microscopy image of fibres prepared with 6% w/v PLA and 4% w/v progesterone; (b) drug release profiles for fibres prepared from solutions of 6% w/v PLA and 2, 4 or 8% progesterone (P4). (Reproduced with permission from Oliveira, J. E.; Medeiros, E. S.; Cardozo, L.; Voll, F.; Madureira, E. H.; Mattoso, L. H.; Assis, O. B. 'Development of poly(lactic acid) nanostructured membranes for the controlled delivery of progesterone to livestock animals.' *Mater. Sci. Eng. C* 33 (2013): 844–849. Copyright Elsevier 2014.)

A study comparing electrospun and solution-blown fibres of poly(3-hydroxybutyrate-co-3-hydroxyvalerate) loaded with sodium diclofenac has also been reported.[26] The drug-loaded fibres were slightly larger in diameter when generated by electrospinning, and the size uniformity was higher through solution blowing. In general there was a greater amount of burst release seen with the electrospun fibres, but otherwise there were no clear trends in the drug release data.

Solution-blown fibres have additionally been created loaded with oil extracted from the medicinal plant *Copaifera* sp., which is often explored for antimicrobial purposes.[28] These materials were constructed from a blend of the polymers PLA and PVP, and were around 1 µm in diameter. An increased PVP content was found to result in increased anti-bacterial activity after 24 h.

The melt blowing process has also received some attention in the pharmaceutical setting, and the fibres produced compared with those from both solution and melt electrospinning.[29] Marosi's team generated formulations from a vinylpyrrolidone–vinyl acetate copolymer, employing poly(ethylene glycol) (PEG) as a plasticiser and carvedilol as a model drug. All three methods led to fibres, with the solution electrospun fibres narrowest (at *ca.* 2 µm in diameter), followed by the melt-blown (10 µm) and melt-spun (50 µm) products. Carvedilol was rendered into the amorphous physical form by all three processing techniques, and all the formulations were able to accelerate the drug dissolution process. The melt-blown and melt electrospun systems led to the fastest release, with almost identical release profiles, while the solution-electrospun fibres freed their drug cargo somewhat more slowly.

A variant of the solution-blowing technique has been applied to the processing of living cells (in this setting it has been referred to as *biothreading*).[30] Using a pressurised coaxial needle with the exterior fluid comprising a viscous polydimethylsiloxane solution and an aqueous cell suspension in the core, cells can be processed into scaffolds with no noticeable loss in viability.

6.6 Electroblowing

Electrospinning and melt/solution blowing can be combined in a process known as electroblowing. This employs both electricity and a gas flow to aid fibre elongation and solidification. The experimental apparatus uses a similar spinneret to that in Figure 6.5, and in addition to the gas flow a potential difference is applied between the spinneret and the collector. This technique has been shown to have significant potential in medical applications: in 2014, Jiang *et al.* applied electroblowing *in vitro* and *in vivo* to deliver a homogeneous and continuous layer of a medical glue to stop bleeding during liver resection.[31]

More recently, Balogh *et al.* prepared fibres of 2-hydroxypropyl-β-cyclodextrin loaded with sodium diclofenac.[32] They found that when electrospinning this system, very frequent clogging of the spinneret occurred. Electroblowing overcame this issue and additionally allowed faster flow rates to be used, increasing the amount of material that could be produced. However, the uniformity of the fibre products was compromised, with more 'beads-on-string' type morphology seen with the blown products. In both cases, the fibres comprised amorphous solid dispersions with no crystalline drug evident. The electroblown fibres dissolved a little more slowly than those from electrospinning, but still much more rapidly than a physical mixture of drug and cyclodextrin.

A subsequent study using Eudragit E and itraconazole (an antifungal active pharmaceutical ingredient) also found that a faster flow rate could be used in blowing, but that the fibre products from the latter had less regular morphologies.[33] Again, the drug was amorphously dispersed in the fibres, and the dissolution profiles of the electrospun and electroblown systems were very similar.

6.7 Pressurised gyration

Pressurised gyration can be regarded as a combination of the centrifugal and blowing approaches. First reported by Mahalingam and Edirisinghe in 2013, it involves a pressurised solution of a polymer being rapidly rotated.[16] The experimental set-up is depicted in Figure 6.7. In essence, it comprises a cylinder with a number of small orifices on its surface. This cylinder is loaded with a polymer solution, which is then pressurised by an inert gas (with pressures up to around 0.3 MPa). The cylinder sits inside a static collector and is rotated at speeds of up to 36,000 rpm. The centrifugal forces and pressure drive the polymer solution out through the orifices, and the solvent rapidly evaporates to produce fibres. The technique has the potential to be very easily scalable, with lab set-ups able to produce up to 6 kg of fibres per hour.[16]

In the initial development of this technique, the polymer PEO was dissolved in water and a range of processing parameters investigated.[16] Through a judicious choice of polymer concentration, applied pressure and rotation rate, the fibre diameter could be varied between around 60 and 1000 nm. The technique has since been extended to a range of polymers,[34] including PVP[35] and blends of carboxymethylcellulose, sodium alginate or polyacrylic acid with PEO.[36] The latter were found to have significant potential as vaginal mucoadhesive formulations.

Pressurised gyration can also be employed to yield drug-loaded fibres.[37] A detailed study of PVP/ibuprofen fibres prepared in this way was performed by Raimi-Abraham *et al.* in 2015.[37] Pure PVP fibres from pressurised hydration had nanoscale diameters, but after inclusion of ibuprofen the fibres were found to become wider, with diameters on the micron scale. Scanning electron microscopy images of the fibres

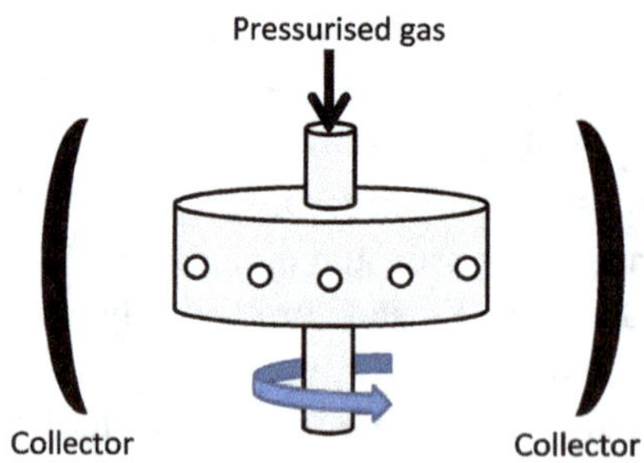

Figure 6.7 A schematic illustration of the experimental apparatus used for centrifugal spinning.

are depicted in Figure 6.8(a) and (b). They comprised amorphous composites of the drug and polymer, and accelerated the dissolution rate of the drug (Figure 6.8(c)). In non-sink conditions, super-saturation could be achieved (Figure 6.8(d)).

Protein active ingredients may also be formulated into fibres using the pressurised gyration route, as has been demonstrated for the gold-binding dodecapeptide Au-BP2.[38] This confirms that the approach is not simply confined to polymers and small molecules, and that complex biomolecules with fragile 3D structures can also be processed.

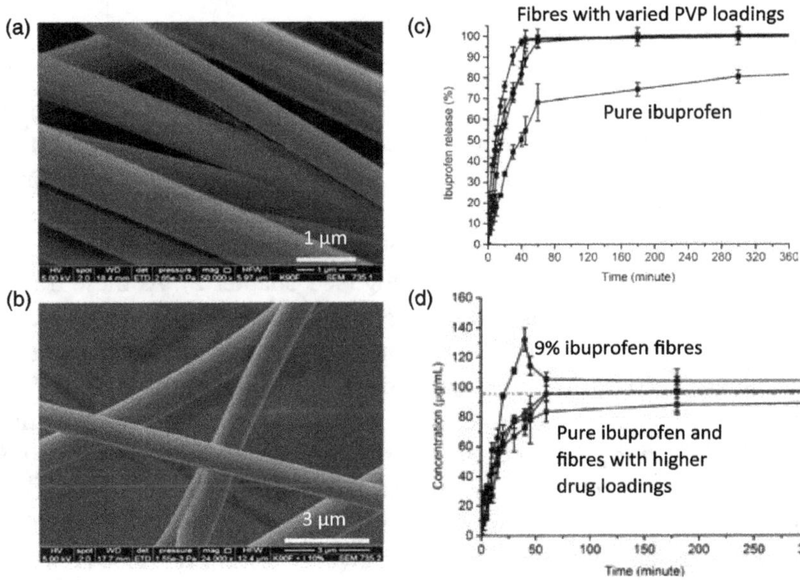

Figure 6.8 Poly(vinyl pyrrolidone) (PVP)–ibuprofen fibres prepared by pressurised gyration. Scanning electron microscopy images of (a) pure PVP fibres and (b) PVP–ibuprofen fibres with a drug loading of 9% w/w, together with drug release profiles under (c) sink and (d) non-sink conditions. In (d), the red line denotes the saturation solubility for ibuprofen, and it is clear that the 9% (w/w) ibuprofen fibres lead to concentrations higher than this in the early stages of the release experiment. (Adapted with permission from Raimi-Abraham, B. T.; Mahalingam, S.; Davies, P. J.; Edirisinghe, M.; Craig, D. Q. 'Development and characterization of amorphous nanofiber drug dispersions prepared using pressurized gyration.' *Mol. Pharm.* 12 (2015): 3851–3861. Copyright American Chemical Society 2015.)

Protein-loaded fibres generated by pressurised gyration have been proposed to have applications in biomineralisation.[39] Fibres have also been prepared incorporating metal nanoparticles, with the aim of producing antibacterial formulations.[40] Most pressurised gyration work has been performed using polymer solutions, but recently it has been shown that the technique can similarly be applied to polymer melts.[41] In the latter study, PCL fibres were prepared loaded with silver nanoparticles, and demonstrated to have antibacterial activity.

6.8 Electrospraying

It would be remiss not to mention the process of electrospraying in the context of this volume. Electrospraying is analogous to the electrospinning process, and uses the same equipment. Rather than producing fibres, however, it yields nano- to micron-sized particles. This is because, rather than ejecting a jet of polymer, the Taylor cone instead emits small droplets in electrospraying (see Chapter 2). As these travel towards the collector the solvent evaporates under the electrical field.

Electrospraying arises when, for instance, the polymer molecular weight is too low and/or the solution too dilute to provide a sufficiently large number of polymer chain entanglements to produce fibres (Figure 6.9). Other than their morphology, the particles from electrospraying are rather similar to the fibres produced in electrospinning. They commonly comprise amorphous solid dispersions, and if made of a fast-dissolving polymer this leads to concomitant enhancement of dissolution rate and solubility. Core/shell and multilayered particles can be prepared by using coaxial and multiaxial spinnerets,[42] as can Janus particles.

As mentioned in section 4.10, there are relatively few reports on parameter optimisation for multi-axial electrospinning. However, there are several informative studies mapping the material and processing parameters for coaxial and multi-axial electrospraying.[43] Given the fact that electrospraying and electrospinning are analogous technologies, the reader may find these reports insightful for guiding material and processing parameter optimisation during multi-axial electrospinning.

An elaborate discussion of the benefits of electrosprayed particles lies outside the scope of this work, and the reader is directed to some recent review articles which discuss these in detail.[44, 45] In general, however, the sprayed particles can deliver the same functional performance as electrospun fibres. There are some caveats though, and

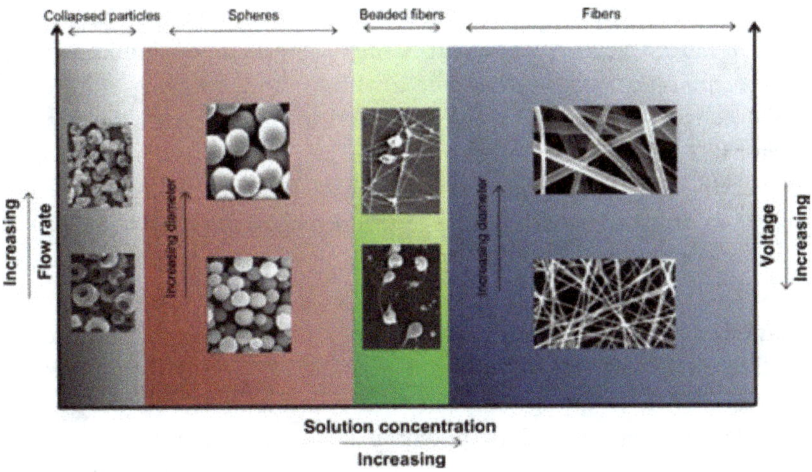

Figure 6.9 A schematic showing the effects of the processing parameters in electrospinning/spraying on the morphology of the products produced. (Reproduced with permission from Zamani, M.; Prabhakaran, M. P.; Ramakrishna, S. 'Advances in drug delivery via electrospun and electrosprayed nanomaterials.' *Int. J. Nanomedicine* 8 (2013): 2997–3017.)

in particular it can be very difficult to recover the particles if collecting them on a standard metal collector. A mat of electrospun fibres is similar to a bowl of spaghetti, in that while the fibres are not covalently linked together they are intertwined and hard to separate. This makes it simple to peel the mat away from the collector. In contrast, no such entanglement exists with electrosprayed particles, and it is common to suffer poor yields as the particles produced adhere strongly to the collector.

Finally, we should note that a number of researchers have explored the combination of electrospinning and electrospraying. The basic idea is to use the fibre mat from electrospinning as a scaffold to provide certain mechanical or physical properties, for instance on which to grow cells or for tissue engineering, and to load this with electrosprayed particles containing a functional component. This can be undertaken either sequentially (spin the scaffold, and then spray particles on to it) or simultaneously (electrospin and spray at the same time). There are a number of examples of both approaches in the literature.

The first report of the combined technique came from Wang *et al.*, who produced a construct for soft-tissue regeneration by simultaneously electrospinning poly(urethane-urea) fibres and spraying core/shell poly(lactic-co-glycolic acid) (PLGA) particles loaded with the growth factor IFG-1.[46] The release rate of the growth factor could be controlled by varying the PLGA concentration and molecular weight, and the composite scaffolds appeared to have good biocompatibility and to be able to promote cell growth.[46]

In another example, a recent study by Zhang's team prepared a scaffold of PCL fibres by electrospinning, and then electrosprayed on to this core/shell PLGA particles containing the protein bovine serum albumin.[47] The resulting composite was found to accelerate the growth of cells, and proposed to have potential in neural regeneration.

Jaworek *et al.* have compared the sequential and simultaneous approaches to assess their efficacy in the coating of Al_2O_3, MgO or TiO_2 nanoparticles on to poly(vinyl chloride), polysulfone or nylon fibres.[48] The simultaneous process was found to lead to a lower-density particle coating, but also a uniform distribution. The sequential approach gave denser layers of particles, but they were localised in the area of the fibre mat which was directly under the needle used for spraying. Thus, in order to ensure even coverage it was necessary to translate the needle or the fibre mat during the collection process.

In another example, Birajdar and Lee have produced fibres which released the embedded drug upon exposure to sonication.[49] To do this, they combined electrospinning and electrospraying to produce core/shell poly(L-lactic acid)/PEO fibres with silica nanoparticles embedded in the shell. This process is illustrated in Figure 6.10(a). Different dyes were incorporated in the two compartments of the fibres to aid visualisation. Immediately after electrospinning, the nanoparticles were loosely attached to the surface of the fibres by weak electrostatic forces, but upon annealing the particles became embedded in the fibres (Figure 6.10(b) and (c)). It was found that the release of rhodamine B from the annealed fibres was much more rapid when sonication was applied (Figure 6.10(d)), thus demonstrating that these materials could be used for drug delivery triggered by sound energy.

The combination of electrospinning and spraying has only recently begun to be explored, and much work remains to be done to understand fully the benefits it can deliver. Two recent review articles discuss the concept in detail, and the interested reader is directed to these for more information.[45d, 50]

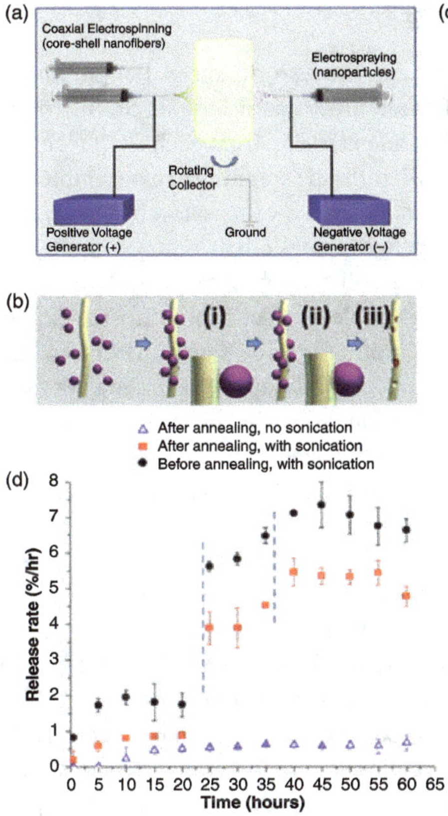

Figure 6.10 Core/shell fibres for sonication-triggered release. (a) The experimental apparatus used to prepare poly(L-lactic acid)/poly(ethylene oxide) fibres with SiO_2 particles on the surface. In essence, this involves the simultaneous electrospinning of the fibres and electrospraying of SiO_2 particles onto the same collector. (b) A schematic showing the release mechanism. (i) Immediately after electrospinning the particles are located on the surface of the fibres, but (ii) solvent vapour annealing causes them to become embedded (bottom). (iii) Sonication frees the embedded particles, exposing pores in the fibre surface through which the drug can escape into solution. (c) Scanning electron microscopy images demonstrating that annealing causes the particles to become embedded in the fibres. (d) Release data for the model drug rhodamine B, located only in the core of the fibres. It is clear that release is markedly faster after bursts of sonication, as denoted by the dashed blue lines. (Reproduced with permission from Birajdar, M. S.; Lee, J. 'Sonication-triggered zero-order release by uncorking core–shell nanofibers.' *Chem. Eng. J.* 288 (2016): 1–8. Copyright Elsevier 2016.)

6.9 Microfluidic spinning

Microfluidic spinning is based on the use of micro (sub-millimetre) channels. A large number of these are located in a single microfluidic chip, and the rate and time of liquid expulsion from each channel are precisely controlled by computer. Microfluidic spinning can be coupled with electrospinning, as described in detail in a recent review by Cheng *et al.*[51] While the productivity of microfluidic methods is a major challenge in scale-up, the technique offers the ability to generate fibres with a high level of complexity not easily achievable by electrospinning. For example, using a digitally programmed microfluidic flow, Kang *et al.* created functional microfibres with continuous spatiotemporal coding along the length of the fibre.[52] The fibres contained varied chemical compositions and topography, and localised bioactive agents.

Microfluidic spinning therefore has the potential to enable very precisely tuneable loading of different drugs into a single fibre, allowing for programmable release in different parts of the body at different times. The technique is beginning to be explored for drug delivery applications. However, the materials used in microfluidics are usually hydrogels (crosslinked polymer networks solvated with water). These often have fast degradation rates and as a result can be unsuitable for the extended release of drugs, particularly small molecules. To help mitigate this problem, Chae *et al.* developed a microfluidic spinning method using an isopropyl alcohol sheath flow with an aqueous alginate core flow.[53] This innovation resulted in nanofibres made of highly ordered alginate molecules. Ahn *et al.* loaded ampicillin into alginate fibres prepared in this manner,[54] and found that the ordered structure delayed fibre degradation, allowing extended-release profile of ampicillin over 7 days.

6.10 Fibre production on the move

Researchers have expended significant effort to miniaturise nanofibre production equipment in order to make it portable. Edirisinghe's group were the first to develop a handheld electrohydrodynamic 'gun', which can be used to produce wound dressings or tissue scaffolds at the site of need.[55] This portable apparatus can be used for both electrospinning and electrospraying, as well as coaxial and multi-axial processes. Jiang *et al.* reported a handheld electroblowing device which could precisely deposit fibres on to wound sites,[31] and as a result achieved rapid cessation of bleeding during liver resection *in vivo*. More recently, a series of battery-operated or self-powered portable sets of electrospinning apparatus have been developed for both solution and melt spinning.[56]

These portable production approaches enable a non-contact application of drug-loaded nanofibres to a patient, thereby minimising the need for manual contact with both the medicine and the treatment site. Such an approach has the potential to help preserve drug integrity, reduce the risk of wound infection and facilitate timely delivery of sophisticated nanofibre-based treatments, since the need to package and transport the product is eliminated. Mouthuy *et al.* analysed the performance of portable electrospinning using a wide range of commonly electrospun materials, and demonstrated that the portable approach can deliver fibre mats of quality comparable to those produced with larger benchtop set-ups.[57] Haik *et al.* explored the use of a portable electrospinning device in wound care, and compared the electrospun dressing with traditional paraffin tulle gras dressings on partial-thickness wounds in pigs.[58] They found no delayed wound healing or signs of infection with either dressing type. The portable apparatus was easy to operate, and could be used to apply different formulations and customisable materials.

6.11 Other techniques

Recently, authors have also begun to explore approaches in which polymerisation and fibre production occur in a single step, preparing a solvent-free mixture of monomers and then expelling these from a spinneret while exposing the jet to, for instance, heat or ultraviolet light to initiate polymerisation.[59] Supercritical CO_2 has also been explored as an alternative to traditional liquid solvents.[60] These techniques have been shown to yield fibres, but have not yet been explored for drug delivery purposes. Their feasibility in this regard is thus not established, but the use of supercritical CO_2 requires the use of high pressures and makes the experimental apparatus required more complex and expensive. *In situ* polymerisation could be more promising, but there is a risk of degradation of the active pharmaceutical ingredient during the process (either through chemical reaction with the monomers, or the heat or ultraviolet light used for polymerisation) which would need to be considered.

Another new technique which has been reported very recently is that of pull spinning.[61] This uses a rotating disc with bristles at its surface, which is fed polymer solution from a syringe. The disc spins very quickly, and as a result a solution jet is formed; this ultimately leads to nanoscale fibres. Pull spinning has yet to be applied to drug delivery but would appear to have significant potential in this area.

Table 6.1 The advantages and disadvantages of the major fibre production approaches considered in this chapter

Technique	*Advantages*	*Disadvantages*
Direct current (DC) electro-spinning	Simple and cheap to set up No use of heat Wide range of literature to build on Many different types of drug delivery system can be produced Can easily be used to make complex architectures Can process a wide variety of fragile active ingredients, including proteins and cells A relatively wide variety of solvents and polymers can be processed Wide range of collector types can be used to align fibres or produce different-shaped scaffolds	Low-throughput batch process – only a few 100 mg of samples per hour can be produced Reproducibly controlling environmental parameters can be difficult, leading to batch-to-batch variation Uses volatile solvents with potential health and safety/ environmental implications
Alternating current electro-spinning	Relatively simple and cheap to establish No use of heat Relatively high throughput (*ca.* eight times greater than DC spinning) Drug delivery performance on a par with products from DC electrospinning	Fibre morphology can be less regular than from DC spinning A reduced range of polymers can be processed Little technological development has been undertaken, making new processes harder to establish Uses volatile solvents with potential health and safety/ environmental implications
Melt electro-spinning	No solvents are used – potentially a greener process than solvent spinning Drug delivery performance on a par with products from DC electrospinning Can offer improved drug delivery performance over solution-spun fibres	Use of heat may cause degradation of labile active ingredients or polymers Apparatus more complex than in solution spinning Fibres have larger diameters than those from solution spinning Little technological development has been undertaken, making new processes harder to establish

Centrifugal spinning	Simple and cheap to set up Can avoid the use of heat/solvent as required Drug delivery performance appears promising Potentially larger-scale than solution electrospinning	Fibres have larger diameters than those from solution spinning Little technological development has been undertaken, making new processes harder to establish Use of one of heat or a volatile solvent is required, which may be problematic for labile drugs (heat) or have safety/ environmental problems (solvent)
Blowing	Simple and cheap to set up Can avoid the use of heat/solvent as required Fibre morphology/uniformity can be as good as or better than from electrospinning Drug delivery performance similar to fibres from solution electrospinning Potentially larger-scale than solution electrospinning Can process cells and other fragile active ingredients in the solution-blowing process	Little technological development has been undertaken, making new processes harder to establish Use of one of heat or a volatile solvent is required, which may be problematic for labile drugs (heat) or have safety/ environmental problems (solvent)
Electroblowing	Can overcome problems with needle clogging experienced in solution electrospinning Higher throughput than standard DC solution electrospinning Drug release behaviour very similar to solution electrospinning	Experimental apparatus somewhat more complex than the separate electrospinning or blowing processes Little technological development has been undertaken, making new processes harder to establish Fibre morphology less uniform than from solution electrospinning Uses volatile solvents with potential health and safety/ environmental implications
Pressurised gyration	Experimental apparatus is relatively simple and easily scalable Fibre diameter can be tuned over a wide range Drug delivery properties are promising, and on a par with those of electrospun fibres Can process fragile active ingredients such as proteins	Relatively little technological development has been undertaken, making new processes harder to establish Fibres possibly wider than those produced by electrospinning Generally uses volatile solvents with potential health and safety/environmental implications

6.12 Conclusions

This chapter has presented a brief overview of the alternative approaches to standard solution electrospinning which can be used to generate drug-loaded fibres. A summary of the advantages and disadvantages of each is given in Table 6.1. Some of the techniques discussed involve the use of heat, which can be problematic with thermally labile active ingredients such as proteins or low-melting-point drugs. However, melt approaches are attractive because they obviate the need for volatile (and thus dangerous) solvents, and the use of plasticisers can reduce the temperatures required for processing. Several of the methods discussed are able to operate continuously and produce larger amounts of fibres than standard lab solution DC electrospinning – for instance, AC spinning and pressurised gyration. They are thus possibly more attractive for industry, since they facilitate scaling up. However, the vast majority of the research undertaken on drug-loaded nanofibres to date has used solution spinning with a DC current, and there are already on the market a number of options for scaling up this process. We will consider these in Chapter 7.

6.13 References

1. Luo, C. J.; Stoyanov, S. D.; Stride, E.; Pelan, E.; Edirisinghe, M. 'Electrospinning versus fibre production methods: From specifics to technological convergence.' *Chem. Soc. Rev.* 41 (2012): 4708–4735.
2. Qi, S.; Craig, D. 'Recent developments in micro- and nanofabrication techniques for the preparation of amorphous pharmaceutical dosage forms.' *Adv. Drug Deliv. Rev.* 100 (2016): 67–84.
3. Kessick, R.; Fenn, J.; Tepper, G. 'The use of AC potentials in electrospraying and electrospinning processes.' *Polymer* 45 (2004): 2981–2984.
4. Sarkar, S.; Deevi, S.; Tepper, G. 'Biased AC electrospinning of aligned polymer nanofibers.' *Macromol. Rapid Commun.* 28 (2007): 1034–1039.
5. Balogh, A.; Cselko, R.; Demuth, B.; Verreck, G.; Mensch, J.; Marosi, G.; Nagy, Z. K. 'Alternating current electrospinning for preparation of fibrous drug delivery systems.' *Int. J. Pharm.* 495 (2015): 75–80.
6. Balogh, A.; Farkas, B.; Verreck, G.; Mensch, J.; Borbas, E.; Nagy, B.; Marosi, G.; Nagy, Z. K. 'AC and DC electrospinning of hydroxypropylmethylcellulose with polyethylene oxides as secondary polymer for improved drug dissolution.' *Int. J. Pharm.* 505 (2016): 159–166.
7. Balogh, A.; Farkas, B.; Palvolgyi, A.; Domokos, A.; Demuth, B.; Marosi, G.; Nagy, Z. K. 'Novel alternating current electrospinning of

hydroxypropylmethylcellulose acetate succinate (HPMCAS) nanofibers for dissolution enhancement: The importance of solution conductivity.' *J. Pharm. Sci.* 106 (2017): 1634–1643.

8. Brown, T. D.; Dalton, P. D.; Hutmacher, D. W. 'Melt electrospinning today: An opportune time for an emerging polymer process.' *Prog. Polym. Sci.* 56 (2016): 116–166.
9. Nagy, Z. K.; Balogh, A.; Dravavolgyi, G.; Ferguson, J.; Pataki, H.; Vajna, B.; Marosi, G. 'Solvent-free melt electrospinning for preparation of fast dissolving drug delivery system and comparison with solvent-based electrospun and melt extruded systems.' *J. Pharm. Sci.* 102 (2013): 508–517.
10. Balogh, A.; Dravavolgyi, G.; Farago, K.; Farkas, A.; Vigh, T.; Soti, P. L.; Wagner, I.; Madarasz, J.; Pataki, H.; Marosi, G.; Nagy, Z. K. 'Plasticized drug-loaded melt electrospun polymer mats: Characterization, thermal degradation, and release kinetics.' *J. Pharm. Sci.* 103 (2014): 1278–1287.
11. Lian, H.; Meng, Z. 'Melt electrospinning vs. solution electrospinning: A comparative study of drug-loaded poly (ε-caprolactone) fibres.' *Mater. Sci. Eng. C* 74 (2017): 117–123.
12. Hochleitner, G.; Jungst, T.; Brown, T. D.; Hahn, K.; Moseke, C.; Jakob, F.; Dalton, P. D.; Groll, J. 'Additive manufacturing of scaffolds with submicron filaments via melt electrospinning writing.' *Biofabrication* 7 (2015): 035002.
13. McCann, J. T.; Marquez, M.; Xia, Y. 'Melt coaxial electrospinning: A versatile method for the encapsulation of solid materials and fabrication of phase change nanofibers.' *Nano Lett.* 6 (2006): 2868–2872.
14. Sarkar, K.; Gomez, C.; Zambrano, S.; Ramirez, M.; de Hoyos, E.; Vasquez, H.; Lozano, K. 'Electrospinning to Forcespinning.' *Mater. Today* 13 (2010): 12–14.
15. Dosunmu, O. O.; Chase, G. G.; Kataphinan, W.; Reneker, D. H. 'Electrospinning of polymer nanofibres from multiple jets on a porous tubular surface.' *Nanotechnology* 17 (2006): 1123–1127.
16. Mahalingam, S.; Edirisinghe, M. 'Forming of polymer nanofibers by a pressurised gyration process.' *Macromol. Rapid Commun.* 34 (2013): 1134–1139.
17. Badrossamay, M. R.; McIlwee, H. A.; Goss, J. A.; Parker, K. K. 'Nanofiber assembly by rotary jet-spinning.' *Nano Lett.* 10 (2010): 2257–2261.
18. Zander, N. E. 'Formation of melt and solution spun polycaprolactone fibers by centrifugal spinning.' *J. Appl. Polym. Sci.* 132 (2015): 41269.
19. Amalorpava Mary, L. 'Centrifugal spun ultrafine fibrous web as a potential drug delivery vehicle.' *Express Polym. Lett.* 7 (2013): 238–248.
20. Buzgo, M.; Rampichova, M.; Vocetkova, K.; Sovkova, V.; Lukasova, V.; Doupnik, M.; Mickova, A.; Rustichelli, F.; Amler, E. 'Emulsion centrifugal spinning for production of 3D drug releasing nanofibres with core/shell structure.' *RSC Adv.* 7 (2017): 1215–1228.

21. Marano, S.; Barker, S. A.; Raimi-Abraham, B. T.; Missaghi, S.; Rajabi-Siahboomi, A.; Craig, D. Q. 'Development of micro-fibrous solid dispersions of poorly water-soluble drugs in sucrose using temperature-controlled centrifugal spinning.' *Eur. J. Pharm. Biopharm.* 103 (2016): 84–94.
22. Zhang, X.; Lu, Y. 'Centrifugal spinning: An alternative approach to fabricate nanofibers at high speed and low cost.' *Polym. Rev.* 54 (2014): 677–701.
23. (a) Kancheva, M.; Toncheva, A.; Manolova, N.; Rashkov, I. 'Advanced centrifugal electrospinning setup.' *Mater. Lett.* 136 (2014): 150–152; (b) Erickson, A. E.; Edmondson, D.; Chang, F. C.; Wood, D.; Gong, A.; Levengood, S. L.; Zhang, M. 'High-throughput and high-yield fabrication of uniaxially-aligned chitosan-based nanofibers by centrifugal electrospinning.' *Carbohydr. Polym.* 134 (2015): 467–474.
24. (a) Liao, C.-C.; Wang, C.-C.; Shih, K.-C.; Chen, C.-Y. 'Electrospinning fabrication of partially crystalline bisphenol A polycarbonate nanofibers: Effects on conformation, crystallinity, and mechanical properties.' *Eur. Polym. J.* 47 (2011): 911–924; (b) Edmondson, D.; Cooper, A.; Jana, S.; Wood, D.; Zhang, M. 'Centrifugal electrospinning of highly aligned polymer nanofibers over a large area.' *J. Mater. Chem.* 22 (2012): 18646–18652.
25. Wang, L.; Chang, M.-W.; Ahmad, Z.; Zheng, H.; Li, J.-S. 'Mass and controlled fabrication of aligned PVP fibers for matrix type antibiotic drug delivery systems.' *Chem. Eng. J.* 307 (2017): 661–669.
26. Souza, M. A.; Sakamoto, K. Y.; Mattoso, L. H. C. 'Release of the diclofenac sodium by nanofibers of poly(3-hydroxybutyrate-co-3-hydroxyvalerate) obtained from electrospinning and solution blow spinning.' *J. Nanomater.* 2014 (2014): 129035.
27. Oliveira, J. E.; Medeiros, E. S.; Cardozo, L.; Voll, F.; Madureira, E. H.; Mattoso, L. H.; Assis, O. B. 'Development of poly(lactic acid) nanostructured membranes for the controlled delivery of progesterone to livestock animals.' *Mater. Sci. Eng. C* 33 (2013): 844–849.
28. Bonan, R. F.; Bonan, P. R.; Batista, A. U.; Sampaio, F. C.; Albuquerque, A. J.; Moraes, M. C.; Mattoso, L. H.; Glenn, G. M.; Medeiros, E. S.; Oliveira, J. E. '*In vitro* antimicrobial activity of solution blow spun poly(lactic acid)/polyvinylpyrrolidone nanofibers loaded with Copaiba (*Copaifera* sp.) oil.' *Mater. Sci. Eng. C* 48 (2015): 372–377.
29. Balogh, A.; Farkas, B.; Farago, K.; Farkas, A.; Wagner, I.; Van Assche, I.; Verreck, G.; Nagy, Z. K.; Marosi, G. 'Melt-blown and electrospun drug-loaded polymer fiber mats for dissolution enhancement: A comparative study.' *J. Pharm. Sci.* 104 (2015): 1767–1776.
30. Arumuganathar, S.; Irvine, S.; McEwan, J. R.; Jayasinghe, S. N. 'A novel direct aerodynamically assisted threading methodology for generating

biologically viable microthreads encapsulating living primary cells.' *J. Appl. Polym. Sci.* 107 (2008): 1215–1225.

31. Jiang, K.; Long, Y. Z.; Chen, Z. J.; Liu, S. L.; Huang, Y. Y.; Jiang, X.; Huang, Z. Q. 'Airflow-directed *in situ* electrospinning of a medical glue of cyanoacrylate for rapid hemostasis in liver resection.' *Nanoscale* 6 (2014): 7792–7798.
32. Balogh, A.; Horváthová, T.; Fülöp, Z.; Loftsson, T.; Harasztos, A. H.; Marosi, G.; Nagy, Z. K. 'Electroblowing and electrospinning of fibrous diclofenac sodium–cyclodextrin complex-based reconstitution injection.' *J. Drug Del. Sci. Technol.* 26 (2015): 28–34.
33. Soti, P. L.; Bocz, K.; Pataki, H.; Eke, Z.; Farkas, A.; Verreck, G.; Kiss, E.; Fekete, P.; Vigh, T.; Wagner, I.; Nagy, Z. K.; Marosi, G. 'Comparison of spray drying, electroblowing and electrospinning for preparation of Eudragit E and itraconazole solid dispersions.' *Int. J. Pharm.* 494 (2015): 23–30.
34. (a) Mahalingam, S.; Raimi-Abraham, B. T.; Craig, D. Q. M.; Edirisinghe, M. 'Solubility–spinnability map and model for the preparation of fibres of polyethylene (terephthalate) using gyration and pressure.' *Chem. Eng. J.* 280 (2015): 344–353; (b) Mahalingam, S.; Ren, G. G.; Edirisinghe, M. J. 'Rheology and pressurised gyration of starch and starch-loaded poly(ethylene oxide).' *Carbohydr. Polym.* 114 (2014): 279–287.
35. Raimi-Abraham, B. T.; Mahalingam, S.; Edirisinghe, M.; Craig, D. Q. 'Generation of poly(*N*-vinylpyrrolidone) nanofibres using pressurised gyration.' *Mater. Sci. Eng. C* 39 (2014): 168–176.
36. Brako, F.; Raimi-Abraham, B.; Mahalingam, S.; Craig, D. Q. M.; Edirisinghe, M. 'Making nanofibres of mucoadhesive polymer blends for vaginal therapies.' *Eur. Polym. J.* 70 (2015): 186–196.
37. Raimi-Abraham, B. T.; Mahalingam, S.; Davies, P. J.; Edirisinghe, M.; Craig, D. Q. 'Development and characterization of amorphous nanofiber drug dispersions prepared using pressurized gyration.' *Mol. Pharm.* 12 (2015): 3851–3861.
38. Zhang, S.; Karaca, B. T.; VanOosten, S. K.; Yuca, E.; Mahalingam, S.; Edirisinghe, M.; Tamerler, C. 'Coupling infusion and gyration for the nanoscale assembly of functional polymer nanofibers integrated with genetically engineered proteins.' *Macromol. Rapid Commun.* 36 (2015): 1322–1328.
39. Wu, X.; Mahalingam, S.; VanOosten, S. K.; Wisdom, C.; Tamerler, C.; Edirisinghe, M. 'New generation of tunable bioactive shape memory mats integrated with genetically engineered proteins.' *Macromol. Biosci.* 17 (2017): 1600270.
40. Illangakoon, U. E.; Mahalingam, S.; Wang, K.; Cheong, Y. K.; Canales, E.; Ren, G. G.; Cloutman-Green, E.; Edirisinghe, M.; Ciric, L. 'Gyrospun

antimicrobial nanoparticle loaded fibrous polymeric filters.' *Mater. Sci. Eng. C* 74 (2017): 315–324.

41. Xu, Z.; Mahalingam, S.; Basnett, P.; Raimi-Abraham, B.; Roy, I.; Craig, D.; Edirisinghe, M. 'Making nonwoven fibrous poly(ε-caprolactone) constructs for antimicrobial and tissue engineering applications by pressurized melt gyration.' *Macromol. Mater. Eng.* 301 (2016): 922–934.
42. (a) Ahmad, Z.; Zhang, H. B.; Farook, U.; Edirisinghe, M.; Stride, E.; Colombo, P. 'Generation of multilayered structures for biomedical applications using a novel tri-needle coaxial device and electrohydrodynamic flow.' *J. R. Soc. Interface.* 5 (2008): 1255–1261; (b) Labbaf, S.; Deb, S.; Cama, G.; Stride, E.; Edirisinghe, M. 'Preparation of multicompartment sub-micron particles using a triple-needle electrohydrodynamic device.' *J. Colloid Interface Sci.* 409 (2013): 245–254; (c) Labbaf, S.; Ghanbar, H.; Stride, E.; Edirisinghe, M. 'Preparation of multilayered polymeric structures using a novel four-needle coaxial electrohydrodynamic device.' *Macromol. Rapid Commun.* 35 (2014): 618–623.
43. (a) Loscertales, I. G.; Barrero, A.; Guerrero, I.; Cortijo, R.; Marquez, M.; Ganan-Calvo, A. M. 'Micro/nano encapsulation via electrified coaxial liquid jets.' *Science* 295 (2002): 1695–1698; (b) Lopez-Herrera, J. M. 'Coaxial jets generated from electrified Taylor cones: Scaling laws.' *Aerosol Sci.* 34 (2003): 535–552; (c) Chen, X.; Jia, L.; Yin, X.; Cheng, J.; Lu, J. 'Spraying modes in coaxial jet electrospray with outer driving liquid.' *Phys. Fluids* 17 (2005): 032101; (d) Mei, F.; Chen, D. R. 'Investigation of compound jet electrospray: Particle encapsulation.' *Phys. Fluids* 19 (2007): 103303.
44. Zamani, M.; Prabhakaran, M. P.; Ramakrishna, S. 'Advances in drug delivery via electrospun and electrosprayed nanomaterials.' *Int. J. Nanomedicine* 8 (2013): 2997–3017.
45. (a) Ciach, T. 'Application of electro-hydro-dynamic atomization in drug delivery.' *J. Drug Del. Sci. Technol.* 17 (2007): 367–375; (b) Yurteri, C. U.; Hartman, R. P. A.; Marijnissen, J. C. M. 'Producing pharmaceutical particles via electrospraying with an emphasis on nano and nano-structured particles: A review.' *KONA Powder Part. J.* 28 (2010): 91–115; (c) Jayasinghe, S. N.; Auguste, J.; Scotton, C. J. 'Platform technologies for directly reconstructing 3D living biomaterials.' *Adv. Mater.* 27 (2015): 7794–7799; (d) Bock, N.; Dargaville, T. R.; Woodruff, M. A. 'Electrospraying of polymers with therapeutic molecules: State of the art.' *Prog. Polym. Sci.* 37 (2012): 1510–1551.
46. Wang, F.; Li, Z.; Tamama, K.; Sen, C. K.; Guan, J. 'Fabrication and characterization of prosurvival growth factor releasing, anisotropic scaffolds for enhanced mesenchymal stem cell survival/growth and orientation.' *Biomacromolecules* 10 (2009): 2609–2618.
47. Zhu, W.; Masood, F.; O'Brien, J.; Zhang, L. G. 'Highly aligned nanocomposite

scaffolds by electrospinning and electrospraying for neural tissue regeneration.' *Nanomedicine* 11 (2015): 693–704.

48. Jaworek, A.; Krupa, A.; Lackowski, M.; Sobczyk, A. T.; Czech, T.; Ramakrishna, S.; Sundarrajan, S.; Pliszka, D. 'Nanocomposite fabric formation by electrospinning and electrospraying technologies.' *J. Electrost.* 67 (2009): 435–438.
49. Birajdar, M. S.; Lee, J. 'Sonication-triggered zero-order release by uncorking core–shell nanofibers.' *Chem. Eng. J.* 288 (2016): 1–8.
50. Guarino, V.; Altobelli, R.; Cirillo, V.; Cummaro, A.; Ambrosio, L. 'Additive electrospraying: A route to process electrospun scaffolds for controlled molecular release.' *Polym. Adv. Technol.* 26 (2015): 1359–1369.
51. Cheng, J.; Jun, Y.; Qin, J.; Lee, S. H. 'Electrospinning versus microfluidic spinning of functional fibers for biomedical applications.' *Biomater.* 114 (2017): 121–143.
52. Kang, E.; Jeong, G. S.; Choi, Y. Y.; Lee, K. H.; Khademhosseini, A.; Lee, S. H. 'Digitally tunable physicochemical coding of material composition and topography in continuous microfibres.' *Nature Mater.* 10 (2011): 877–883.
53. Chae, S.-K.; Kang, E.; Khademhosseini, A.; Lee, S.-H. 'Micro/nanometer-scale fiber with highly ordered structures by mimicking the spinning process of silkworm.' *Adv. Mater.* 25 (2013): 3071–3078.
54. Ahn, S. Y.; Mun, C. H.; Lee, S. H. 'Microfluidic spinning of fibrous alginate carrier having highly enhanced drug loading capability and delayed release profile.' *RSC Adv.* 5 (2015): 15172–15181.
55. Sofokleous, P.; Stride, E.; Bonfield, W.; Edirisinghe, M. 'Design, construction and performance of a portable handheld electrohydrodynamic multi-needle spray gun for biomedical applications.' *Mater. Sci. Eng. C* 33 (2013): 213–223.
56. (a) Qin, C. C.; Duan, X. P.; Wang, L.; Zhang, L. H.; Yu, M.; Dong, R. H.; Yan, X.; He, H. W.; Long, Y. Z. 'Melt electrospinning of poly(lactic acid) and polycaprolactone microfibers by using a hand-operated Wimshurst generator.' *Nanoscale* 7 (2015): 16611–16615; (b) Xu, S. C.; Qin, C. C.; Yu, M.; Dong, R. H.; Yan, X.; Zhao, H.; Han, W. P.; Zhang, H. D.; Long, Y. Z. 'A battery-operated portable handheld electrospinning apparatus.' *Nanoscale* 7 (2015): 12351–12355; (c) Yan, X.; Yu, M.; Zhang, L. H.; Jia, X. S.; Li, J. T.; Duan, X. P.; Qin, C. C.; Dong, R. H.; Long, Y. Z. 'A portable electrospinning apparatus based on a small solar cell and a hand generator: Design, performance and application.' *Nanoscale* 8 (2016): 209–213.
57. Mouthuy, P.-A.; Groszkowski, L.; Ye, H. 'Performances of a portable electrospinning apparatus.' *Biotechnol. Lett.* 37 (2015): 1107–1116.
58. Haik, J.; Kornhaber, R.; Blal, B.; Harats, M. 'The feasibility of a handheld electrospinning device for the application of nanofibrous wound dressings.' *Adv. Wound Care* 6 (2017): 166–174.

59. Zhang, B.; Yan, X.; He, H.-W.; Yu, M.; Ning, X.; Long, Y.-Z. 'Solvent-free electrospinning: Opportunities and challenges.' *Polym. Chem.* 8 (2017): 333–352.
60. Levit, N.; Tepper, G. 'Supercritical CO_2-assisted electrospinning.' *J. Supercrit. Fluids* 31 (2004): 329–333.
61. Deravi, L. F.; Sinatra, N. R.; Chantre, C. O.; Nesmith, A. P.; Yuan, H.; Deravi, S. K.; Goss, J. A.; MacQueen, L. A.; Badrossamy, M. R.; Gonzalez, G. M.; Phillips, M. D.; Parker, K. K. 'Design and fabrication of fibrous nanomaterials using pull spinning.' *Macromol. Mater. Eng.* 302 (2017): 1600404.

7

From Theory to Practice

7.1 Introduction

The previous chapters have enumerated the range of electrospinning approaches which can be implemented, and explored how the fibres thereby produced can be applied in drug delivery, as well as briefly introducing a range of other fibre production techniques. However, at the time of writing there are no electrospun fibre-based pharmaceutical products on the market, despite the distinct promise of the approach. This is because there are a large number of hurdles lying between exciting results obtained in the lab and being able to produce formulations in the commercial environment. We will discuss these in this chapter.

7.2 Scale-up

The standard lab electrospinning apparatus works at somewhere between 0.5 and 20 ml h^{-1}, and thus in a day of spinning at most some 200 ml of fluid can be processed. With a typical polymer concentration of around 10% w/v, this amounts to a maximum daily yield of 20 g of fibres – clearly a long way from the kilograms or tonnes per day required for an industrial process. The ability to produce fibres in much larger quantities is thus required, which necessitates that modifications be made to the experimental equipment. In order to scale up the electrospinning process, attention must be paid to two key components of the apparatus: the spinneret and the collector.

7.2.1 The spinneret

The design of the spinneret has been discussed in some detail previously (sections 2.6.3, 3.2.3 and 4.2.3), but in essence in most cases it comprises a flat-tipped metal needle. The earliest attempts to scale up the electrospinning process aimed to achieve this by simply using multiple needles and feeding these from a single reservoir of polymer solution. These can be arranged in a linear or circular manner (Figure 7.1).[1]

In order to generate fibres on a sufficiently large scale for commercial production, however, the number of needles required is very high: of the order of thousands. The Toptec company has produced apparatus which works on this principle, with the needles ejecting solution upwards (contrary to the usual protocol in lab-based experiments, which spin horizontally or downwards) to avoid any polymer droplets falling on to the collector from the nozzles.[2] Inovenso also use a multi-nozzle approach in their commercial-scale spinning equipment.[3] A number of problems exist with the multi-needle approach, however. The reliability of the process is often sub-optimal, and issues of needle clogging and other machine maintenance difficulties frequently arise. The consistency and reproducibility of the product can also be challenging to ensure.

One of the key issues with the multi-needle approach is that the electric field around a given needle is affected by the presence of other electrospinning jets in its vicinity, which can result in inhomogeneity in the products.[4] This can be ameliorated to an extent by the use of auxiliary or secondary electrodes.[5] Other researchers have successfully used a hollow tube with holes drilled in the side as a replacement for multiple needles,[6] which makes for a simpler structure. The channels of a microfluidic chip can also be used to this end.[7] However, the problems caused by adjacent jets interfering with one another are still present in these cases.

A more robust solution to the issues of clogging and field inhomogeneity is to implement a needle-free process. Rather than ejecting a

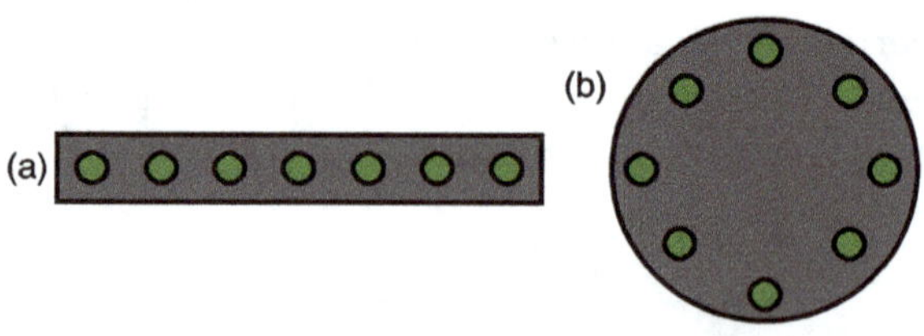

Figure 7.1 Different arrangements of needles in multi-needle electrospinning, showing (a) linear and (b) circular configurations.

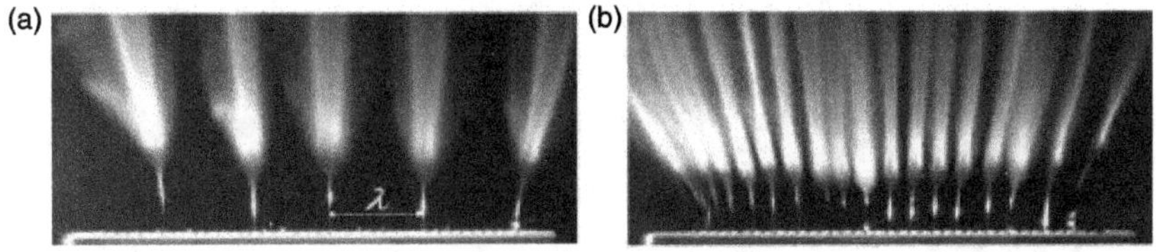

Figure 7.2 Needleless electrospinning of poly(vinyl alcohol) at (a) 32 and (b) 43 kV. (Reproduced with permission from Petrik, S., 'Industrial production technology for nanofibers.' In *Nanofibers – Production, Properties and Functional Applications*, edited by Lin, T., 3–16. Rijeka)

liquid through a needle, this uses an electric field to form a polymer jet from the surface of a liquid. This works in a similar way to standard electrospinning, except that an extended area of a polymer solution's surface is charged. This causes Coulombic repulsions, as described in section 2.4, the formation of a large number of Taylor cones on the surface, and as a result the emission of numerous polymer jets (Figure 7.2).

Needleless electrospinning removes the possibility of clogging, but other challenges arise, because this process is likely to deposit large droplets as well as or instead of fibres. Specialised equipment is needed to ameliorate these challenges, such as the Nanospider technology developed by Elmarco.[8] The original iteration of this equipment used a charged metal cylinder as the fibre generator. The cylinder is partially immersed into a polymer solution and rotated, ensuring that a thin layer of polymer solution coats the top of the cylinder (Figure 7.3). When an electrical current is applied, this results in the emission of a large number of liquid jets upwards from the top of the solution-covered cylinder (Figure 7.3). Higher voltages than in the standard spinning process are typically required (approximately 30–120 kV for free-surface spinning, *cf.* 5–20 kV for needle spinning).[2] The jets which form are distributed across the electrode in the most energetically stable configuration possible. This is in sharp contrast to the multi-needle approach, where the needles are placed by human design. While modelling and calculations can help researchers to design efficient multi-needle spinnerets, the needle-free approach achieves an optimum distribution of Taylor cones without requiring any such modelling. The Nanospider is able to produce up to 50 million m^2 of fibres per year.

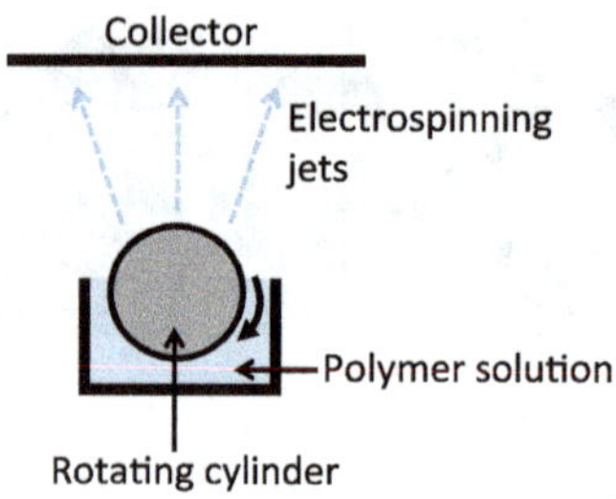

Figure 7.3 The rotating drum electrode used in the Nanospider needleless electrospinning technology.

The rotating drum approach is not the only type of free-surface electrospinning process, and others have reported using magnetic particles,[9] wires,[10] rings,[11] discs,[12] rods[13] and balls[12a] or a fluid-filled bowl as the spinneret.[14] The latter approach uses the edge of the bowl as the spinneret, termed 'edge electrospinning'. These types of free-surface spinning can effectively resolve the problems of fibre inhomogeneity and needle clogging. However, there remain some concerns, because electrospinning typically works with volatile solvents with high vapour pressure, and thus there is a risk of solvent evaporation occurring independently of the electric field. In extreme cases, there is an explosion risk with a large uncovered container of polymer solution being used for spinning.

Several teams of researchers have sought innovative solutions to reduce the exposed solution surface area. This can be achieved by, for instance, dropping the polymer solution slowly from a syringe on to the roller spinneret.[15] In a slightly different approach, Lu *et al.* employed a rotating cone electrode (Figure 7.4), onto which a polymer solution was steadily delivered.[16] This reduced the exposed area, and the method could produce fibres on the 10 g min^{-1} scale, some 1000-fold higher than standard lab electrospinning. Other scientists have used an angled flat plate as the spinneret.[17]

The dropwise addition of polymer solution, angled plate or rotating cone arrangements can solve the problem of exposing a large area of solution, but it can be difficult to control the delivery of polymer to the spinneret and to ensure that this is even and at a constant rate. These approaches have gained traction with industry as well as in the research laboratory, however. Elmarco have, in the newer generations of the Nanospider technology, moved away from a rotating drum set-up to use a static wire continuously coated with a polymer solution as the spinneret (Figure 7.5).[18]

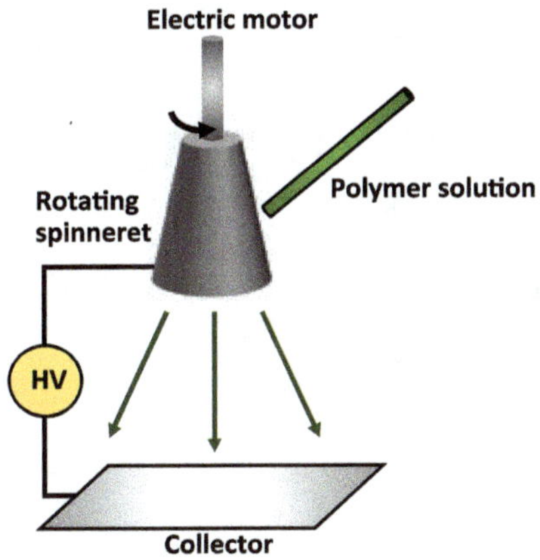

Figure 7.4 The rotating cone methodology used by Lu *et al.*[16] HV: high voltage.

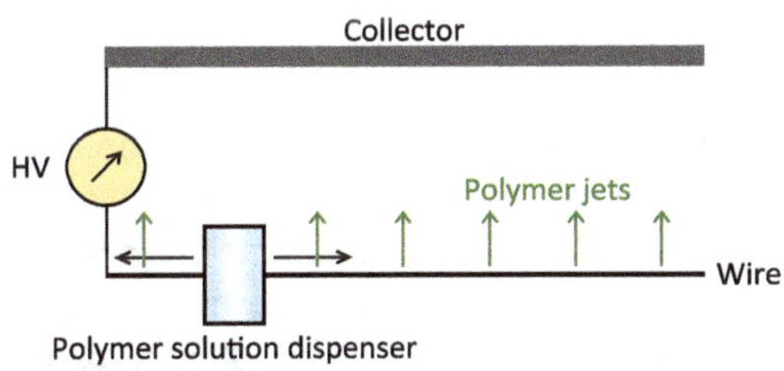

Figure 7.5 Surface electrospinning from a static wire. The wire is charged, and a polymer solution dispenser moves up and down the length of the wire, ensuring that all parts of it are continuously supplied with polymer. HV: high voltage.

Recent work by Molnar and Nagy has developed a novel technique to permit high-throughput spinning while minimising the surface area of solvent exposed to the environment.[19] This uses a corona spinneret, in which the polymer solution can escape from its reservoir via a narrow circular gap, as depicted in Figure 7.6. The spinneret is rotated, and fed continuously with polymer solution. Taylor cones are generated at the edge of the corona when an electrical current is applied. This approach has the advantage of the free-surface approach, in that the positions of the Taylor cones are determined by the properties of the system being spun and the electrospinning parameters, and the cones will thus automatically be arranged in the most stable configuration. The corona spinneret allowed

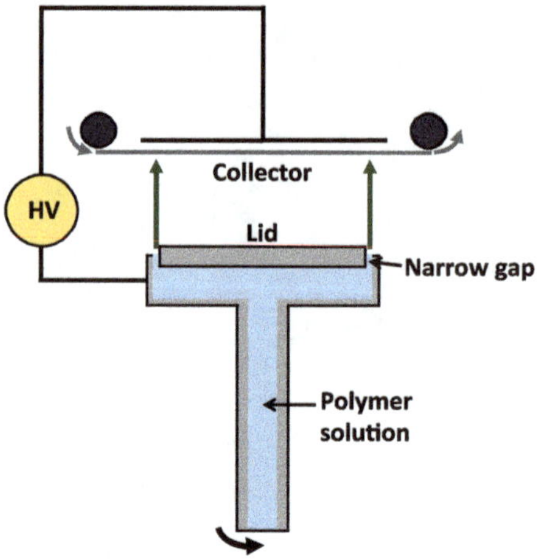

Figure 7.6 The corona approach to high-speed electrospinning reported by Molnar and Nagy.[19] The collector comprises a moving conveyor belt. HV: high voltage.

electrospinning to be performed without any manual intervention for many hours. When poly(vinyl pyrrolidone) and poly(acrylonitrile) (PAN) fibres were prepared with both the standard single-needle and the corona approach, these were almost indistinguishable in their morphologies, although the PAN fibres were slightly narrower when prepared through corona spinning.

Since much of the work to scale up electrospinning has only begun in recent years, the majority of studies have considered the single-fluid process. However, coaxial spinning can also be scaled up, as demonstrated by Wu *et al.*[20] These authors essentially used the multi-needle approach, but rather than having needles protruding from a surface, they nested them inside a block such that the ends of the needles were flat with the edge of the mount. Core/shell fibres with sizes very close to those from a standard coaxial needle were obtained.

The free-surface spinning methodology can also be used to prepare core/shell structures, as reported by Forward *et al.*[10] This study featured a system of two immiscible solutions, one layered on top of another. A wire electrode is raised upwards through these, generating a two-layer coating on the wires, as shown in Figure 7.7. The application of a voltage causes two-compartment Taylor cones to form on the wire surface and polymer jets to be emitted, ultimately yielding core/shell fibres. A rotating spindle of wires was used to produce fibres in a continuous manner.

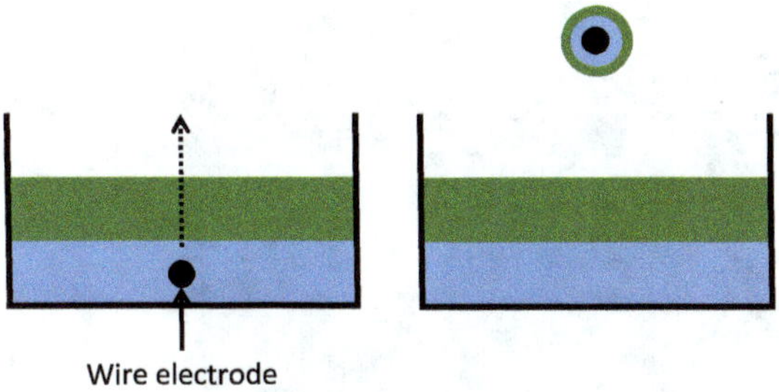

Figure 7.7 Using free-surface electrospinning from wire electrodes to generate core/shell fibres, as reported by Forward *et al.*[10] Two immiscible liquids are placed in a container, and the wire electrode is drawn up through these (left), thereby creating a bilayer of fluids around the electrode (right). Application of an electrical field results in the formation of a compound Taylor cone and thus core/shell fibres are produced.

This approach is potentially a powerful one, but is limited because it requires the two fluids involved to have low miscibility. This limitation can be overcome, and coaxial fibre production successfully scaled up to production rates of around 1 l h^{-1}, using a 'slit surface' method.[21] This is shown in Figure 7.8. In essence, in this approach the two working fluids flow through separate channels but are brought together at a surface as they pass through the exit slits. The application of a high voltage results in compound Taylor cones forming, and thus the production of core/shell fibres. A similar approach, using a polymer bilayer and a 'weir' spinneret, has been demonstrated by Vysloužilová *et al.* to be capable of generating core/shell fibres.[22] Janus fibres may also be produced via a similar needleless route.[23]

Emulsion spinning has also been successfully scaled up via a free-surface strategy, by feeding an emulsion between two parallel, charged, copper wires.[24] Similar, unconfined, approaches can be applied to melt electrospinning. This has been reported by Wang *et al.*, who melted polyethylene on a heated plate and then applied an electric field between this and a collector.[25] This resulted in the formation of 'fingering perturbations' at the edge of the plate, and these in turn emitted polymer jets and generated fibres. Needleless alternating current electrospinning has also been reported.[26] Furthermore, as was noted in Chapter 6 (sections 6.4 and 6.7) the approaches of centrifugal spinning and pressurised gyration are additionally amenable to scale up.[27]

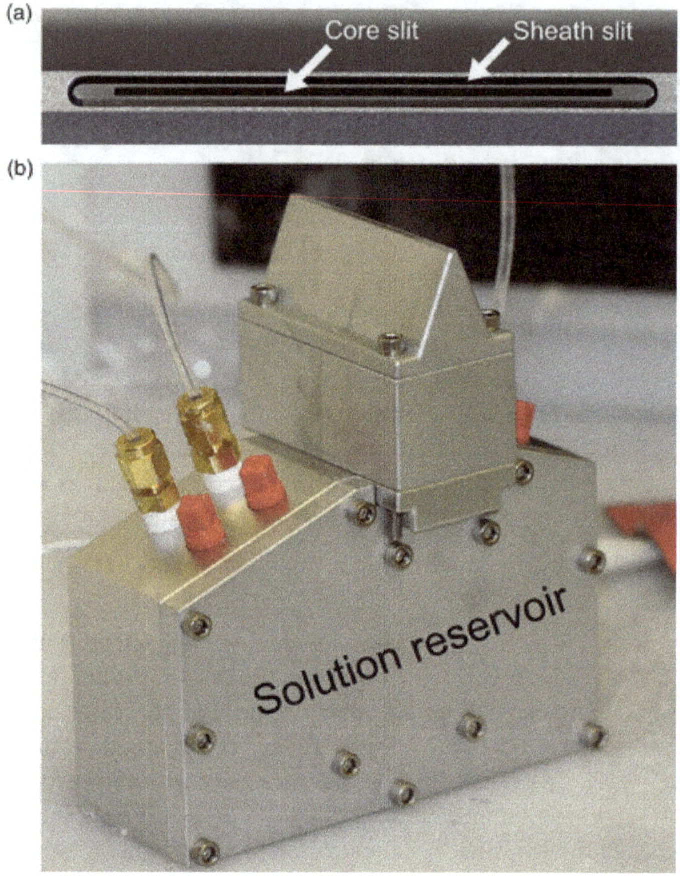

Figure 7.8 The experimental apparatus used in the slit-surface spinning free-surface method, which permits core–shell fibres to be produced on the large scale. The arrangement of slits is shown in (a), and the complete apparatus in (b). (Reproduced with permission from Yan, X.; Marini, J.; Mulligan, R.; Deleault, A.; Sharma, U.; Brenner, M. P.; Rutledge, G. C.; Freyman, T.; Pham, Q. P. 'Slit-surface electrospinning: A novel process developed for high-throughput fabrication of core–sheath fibers.' *PLoS ONE* 10 (2015): e0125407. Copyright Yan *et al.* 2015.)

7.2.2 The collector

In most lab-scale experiments, the collector is simply a flat grounded surface, often a sheet of metal wrapped in aluminium foil. This is perfectly adequate for the majority of experiments, and has the advantages of cost-effectiveness and simplicity. In more advanced set-ups, researchers have used rotating mandrels or parallel electrodes as the collectors to align the fibres produced (section 2.6.4). All of these, however, are inherently batch processes. There is a limit to the amount of fibres which can be collected in one experiment, because as the layer of material on the collector gets thicker the grounding is lost. For scale-up, a continuous process is required, which demands a different collector. This is usually a moving surface or conveyor belt set-up (Figure 7.6).[1, 28] Such collector geometries can both achieve fibre alignment, if desired, and hugely aid the translation to industrial-scale continuous processes.

7.2.3 Safety and environmental considerations

On the lab scale, when processing a few millilitres of liquid per hour, venting the evaporated solvent into the air in the laboratory is probably not a concern with the majority of solvents, and if required a fume cupboard can be used to handle the vapour produced safely. When working on the scale of many litres per hour, however, there is a risk to the safety of the users operating the equipment from high concentrations of solvent in the air, and additionally an ignition risk. Thus, such procedures must take place with the evaporated solvent effectively extracted from the local environment through a robust ventilation system. A range of options exist for doing this, and commercial suppliers such as Nanospider and IME can already provide such systems.

The environment outside the production facility should also be considered, as should wastage. It is not environmentally friendly to vent large volumes of solvent to the atmosphere and then use fresh solvent for subsequent manufacturing, and thus it is desirable to establish facilities which can collect the evaporated solvent, condense it and reuse it in a later spinning process. Venting solvents is tightly regulated by legislation, and robust measures will be required to ensure any facility complies with these.

7.2.4 Scale-up in electrospun drug delivery systems: preliminary studies

A few groups have in recent years begun to compare the drug delivery properties of fibres prepared by standard single-needle and high-speed (scaled-up) electrospinning. Krogstad and Woodrow have undertaken such a study looking to scale up the production of poly(vinyl alcohol) fibres loaded with tenofovir, an antiretroviral drug.[29] The intended application here was as a topical vaginal microbicide for anti-human immunodeficiency virus (HIV) treatment. Free-surface high-throughput spinning was undertaken using Nanospider apparatus fitted with parallel wire electrodes. The fibre properties were very similar regardless of production method, with those from the wire apparatus slightly narrower in diameter than the fibres produced on standard lab equipment. The stability and drug release properties were almost identical from both approaches. However, while the single-needle spinning yielded around 43–135 mg h^{-1} of product, the Nanospider could produce in the region of 2.9–7.7 g h^{-1}, an increase of around 60–70-fold in production capacity.

In other work, Nagy and colleagues have prepared fibres of poly(vinyl pyrrolidone/vinyl acetate) (PVPVA) loaded with the antifungal drug itraconazole using their corona spinneret with a conveyor-belt collector.[30] In the single-needle experiment, they could work with a flow rate of 20 ml h^{-1}, corresponding to 6 g h^{-1} of solid material being produced. The high-speed approach permitted a flow rate of 1500 ml h^{-1} to be realised, yielding 450 g of material every hour: a 75-fold increase. The high-speed fibres had more bead-on-string morphology visible (Figure 7.9(a)–(d)), but in both cases the drug was amorphously distributed in the fibres and drug release was markedly faster than the dissolution of the raw material or a PVPVA/itraconazole cast film, as can be seen in Figure 7.9(e). The resultant fibres could be processed into tablets.[31]

The long-term stability of electrospun formulations will be crucial to successful clinical applications, and the relative stabilities of analogous formulations from high-throughput and standard single-needle spinning have been compared.[32] Fibres were prepared comprising PVPVA or hydroxypropylmethylcellulose (HPMC) as the carrier polymer and itraconazole as a model drug. As noted above, the PVPVA-based fibres prepared in the high-speed approach contained more beads than those from single-fluid spinning, but all consisted of amorphous solid dispersions of drug in polymer. They were stable for 1 year when kept under sealed conditions at 25°C and 60% relative humidity (RH), but when stored in open containers at 40°C and 75% RH, phase separation of the drug and polymer and drug recrystallisation were observed after 3 months. The dissolution profiles of those stored at 25°C/60% RH were indistinguishable from the fresh materials, showing markedly accelerated dissolution over a drug/polymer physical mixture. In contrast, those stored at 40°C/75% RH showed much slower dissolution owing to the recrystallisation of drug, exhibiting behaviour closer to the physical mixture. The high-speed spinning samples were slightly slower to dissolve than those from the single-needle spinning.

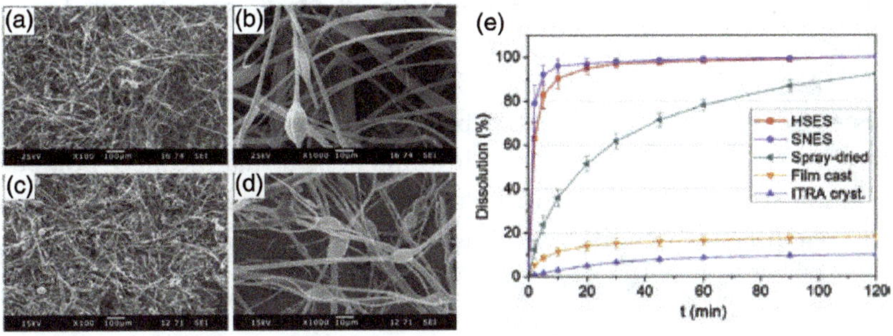

Figure 7.9 A comparison of single-needle and high-speed corona electrospinning for the preparation of poly(vinyl pyrrolidone/vinyl acetate)/itraconazole (ITRA) fibres. Scanning electron microscopy images of (a) and (b) the single-needle fibres, and (c) and (d) the high-speed fibres are shown together with (e) dissolution profiles of high-speed electrospinning (HSES) and single-needle electrospinning (SNES) fibres, compared with analogous spray-dried or film-cast formulations and the raw material. (Adapted with permission from Nagy, Z. K.; Balogh, A.; Demuth, B.; Pataki, H.; Vigh, T.; Szabo, B.; Molnar, K.; Schmidt, B. T.; Horak, P.; Marosi, G.; Verreck, G.; Van Assche, I.; Brewster, M. E. 'High speed electrospinning for scaled-up production of amorphous solid dispersion of itraconazole.' *Int. J. Pharm.* 480 (2015): 137–142. Copyright Elsevier 2015.)

In the case of HPMC, no recrystallisation was observed even after 12 months' storage at 40°C and 75% RH, but it was thought that some changes in the conformations of the drug and polymer occurred during this time since the dissolution rate was slower after storage. As for PVPVA, the dissolution rate of the high-speed spun fibres was slower than for the single-needle fibres, but 100% dissolution inside 2 h was still observed. Here, the stored samples behaved much more similarly to the fresh samples, owing to the lack of phase separation.

Scale-up has also been explored in the case of protein drugs.[33] Poly(vinyl alcohol) or poly(vinyl pyrrolidone) (PVP) fibres loaded with the enzyme β-galactosidase (lactase), widely used for the treatment of lactose intolerance, were generated. Experiments were initially performed on standard lab equipment, and then subsequently using the corona spinning approach. To avoid denaturation of the enzyme, water was employed as the solvent, requiring high voltages of 30 kV for successful spinning. Only minimal (< 5%) loss of enzyme activity was seen with PVP, and the fibres produced on the large scale behaved very similarly to the small-scale batches.

Although the scaled-up production of electrospun drug delivery systems has only begun to be explored very recently, the preliminary results are very encouraging, and it would appear that the large number of small-scale lab studies which have been performed to date have very real potential to be translated to the industrial setting.

7.3 Regulatory requirements and GMP manufacturing

The path to taking a medicine to market is necessarily a long and rather bureaucratic one, since a large number of safeguards are required to ensure patient safety. Each jurisdiction will have its own regulatory body responsible for approving the sale of a new formulation (in the UK, this is the European Medicines Agency (EMA) for products centrally authorised in the European Union and the Medicines and Healthcare products Health Regulatory Agency (MHRA) for nationally authorised products). That said, although the precise procedures to be followed will differ from place to place, the principal stages of taking a medicinal product from the lab to the clinic are similar worldwide, and increasingly harmonised through the procedures of the International Conference on Harmonisation (ICH).[34] For instance, today manufacturers typically control impurities in active pharmaceutical ingredients and validate analytical methods worldwide based on ICH guidelines (which cover the USA, Europe and Japan).

To obtain regulatory approval, the synthetic chemistry behind the active ingredient must be well established, and its chemical structure, stereochemistry, phase purity and impurity profile confirmed using appropriate analytical techniques. A robust manufacturing process must be in place, with appropriate in-process controls to ensure that all products meet the required quality standards. The efficacy and safety of the drug, and the formulation, must be demonstrated *in vitro*, *in vivo* in animals and in clinical trials. The stability of the formulation and its shelf-life must be established and appropriate specifications established. These processes are complex, expensive and time-consuming, but all are carried out efficiently and successfully by a number of companies worldwide, and thus all aspects of the regulatory framework which can be directly translated to fibre products should be relatively straightforward to implement. In the view of the authors, the major difference between a fibre product and one prepared in more conventional ways – for instance, through spray or freeze drying – lies in the manufacturing process, and thus here is where the major challenge to translation lies.

We have discussed above the requirement to produce large amounts of material, and it is clear that a number of plausible routes to scale-up exist. Making large volumes of material is not sufficient, however, and attention must also be paid to the quality and reproducibility of the formulations generated. For use in medical products, ultimately it will be necessary to perform electrospinning under good manufacturing practice (GMP) guidelines. GMP covers a range of aspects of a pharmaceutical manufacturing process, including the development, manufacture, packaging and testing of the product. It takes into consideration the premises used for manufacture, the personnel involved, the different steps of the production process and the quality management systems in place to assure product quality. Robust training regimes are required, as well as procedures for dealing with out-of-specification events, complaints and product recall. Thorough documentation must be produced, with a traceable audit trail for every batch of product generated.

A detailed discussion of GMP lies outside the scope of this chapter. In essence, however, GMP ensures that products of the appropriate quality are consistently produced and controlled, and that manufactured materials and products comply with standards appropriate for their intended use as enforced by the appropriate regulatory authority (e.g. the EMA or MHRA). For instance, it is vital to ensure that the product contains the correct drug at the appropriate strength, that impurities and microbial content are controlled, and where appropriate that the drug is released at a pre-determined rate. The product must be packaged properly and protected against degradation or damage, and be correctly labelled. This is ensured by putting in place a pharmaceutical quality system which incorporates the requirements of GMP and quality risk management. The interested reader may find the EU and UK GMP guidelines helpful to understand the requirements in more detail.[35]

In essence, therefore, to meet GMP requirements it will be necessary to produce large batches of electrospun fibres reproducibly with consistent properties and performance between batches. This is currently a problem because, although parameters such as temperature and RH can be precisely controlled through bespoke systems such as those produced by IME Technologies,[36] these are expensive and to date there has been little convergence between precise control of the process and scale-up (i.e. it has been possible to produce relatively small amounts of fibres with a very high level of control, or large amounts of materials with less control, but not both). That said, Elmarco now produce an air-conditioning attachment for their industrial apparatus to permit precise control of the environmental parameters, and these types of innovations can be expected to accelerate in the coming years.

To ensure product quality, in addition to controlling the processing parameters, some form of inline (i.e. live, in real time) monitoring of product quality will be required to ensure that if there are any problems during production they can be rapidly detected, and production halted until the issues have been addressed. The use of a volatile solvent in electrospinning is also potentially problematic. Environmental regulations must be considered in the disposal of the solvent, and processes established to ensure that any residual solvent in the final products falls below acceptable limits.

Although challenging, electrospinning is no more complex than standard industry processes such as hot melt extrusion or spray drying (see section 1.5), and thus undertaking it under GMP conditions should be eminently achievable. This is shown by a report in the literature,[37] which placed Nanospider apparatus in a clean room operated to GMP conditions and generated fibres to be used as an artificial extracellular matrix for stem cell applications. Further, the UK-based Electrospinning Company also routinely performs electrospinning under GMP conditions using a clean room.[38]

7.4 Conclusions

In this chapter, we have briefly reviewed the further steps which need to be taken to translate the wide range of promising fibre formulations which have been prepared in the research laboratory to the clinic. Although there remain challenges and obstacles to overcome, the main barriers comprise the need to produce large amounts of materials in a reproducible and quality-controlled environment, and to move the products through the various stages of development towards regulatory approval. As has been discussed, there is still work to do in terms of the former, but very significant steps forward have been made in recent years. Pharmaceutical companies have a tremendous weight of experience in the latter, and thus it is to be expected that fibre-based drug delivery systems will have an excellent chance of making their way to the clinic in the relatively near future.

7.5 References

1. Persano, L.; Camposeo, A.; Tekmen, C.; Pisignano, D. 'Industrial upscaling of electrospinning and applications of polymer nanofibers: A review.' *Macromol. Mater. Eng.* 298 (2013): 504–520.
2. Petrik, S., 'Industrial production technology for nanofibers.' In *Nanofibers – Production, Properties and Functional Applications*, edited by Lin, T., 3–16. Rijeka: InTech, 2011.
3. http://inovenso.com/about/. Accessed 26 June 2017.
4. Theron, S. A.; Yarin, A. L.; Zussman, E.; Kroll, E. 'Multiple jets in electrospinning: Experiment and modeling.' *Polymer* 46 (2005): 2889–2899.
5. Kim, G. H.; Cho, Y. S.; Kim, W. D. 'Stability analysis for multi-jets electrospinning process modified with a cylindrical electrode.' *Eur. Polym. J.* 42 (2006): 2031–2038.
6. Varabhas, J. S.; Chase, G. G.; Reneker, D. H. 'Electrospun nanofibers from a porous hollow tube.' *Polymer* 49 (2008): 4226–4229.
7. Srivastava, Y.; Marquez, M.; Thorsen, T. 'Multijet electrospinning of conducting nanofibers from microfluidic manifolds.' *J. Appl. Polym. Sci.* 106 (2007): 3171–3178.
8. www.elmarco.com/. Accessed 26 June 2017.
9. Yarin, A. L.; Zussman, E. 'Upward needleless electrospinning of multiple nanofibers.' *Polymer* 45 (2004): 2977–2980.
10. Forward, K. M.; Flores, A.; Rutledge, G. C. 'Production of core/shell fibers by electrospinning from a free surface.' *Chem. Eng. Sci.* 104 (2013): 250–259.
11. Wang, X.; Lin, T.; Wang, X. 'Scaling up the production rate of nanofibers by needleless electrospinning from multiple ring.' *Fiber. Polym.* 15 (2014): 961–965.
12. (a) Niu, H.; Wang, X.; Lin, T. 'Needleless electrospinning: Influences of fibre generator geometry.' *J. Text. I.* 103 (2012): 787–794; (b) Niu, H.; Lin, T.; Wang, X. 'Needleless electrospinning. I. A comparison of cylinder and disk nozzles.' *J. Appl. Polym. Sci.* 114 (2009): 3524–3530.
13. Wu, D.; Xiao, Z.; Teh, K. S.; Han, Z.; Luo, G.; Shi, C.; Sun, D.; Zhao, J.; Lin, L. 'High-throughput rod-induced electrospinning.' *J. Phys. D.* 49 (2016): 365302.
14. Thoppey, N. M.; Gorga, R. E.; Clarke, L. I.; Bochinski, J. R. 'Control of the electric field–polymer solution interaction by utilizing ultra-conductive fluids.' *Polymer* 55 (2014): 6390–6398.
15. Tang, S.; Zeng, Y.; Wang, X. 'Splashing needleless electrospinning of nanofibres.' *Polym. Sci. Eng.* 50 (2010): 2252–2257.
16. Lu, B.; Wang, Y.; Liu, Y.; Duan, H.; Zhou, J.; Zhang, Z.; Wang, Y.; Li, X.; Wang, W.; Lan, W.; Xie, E. 'Superhigh-throughput needleless electrospinning using a rotary cone as spinneret.' *Small* 6 (2010): 1612–1616.

17. Thoppey, N. M.; Bochinski, J. R.; Clarke, L. I.; Gorga, R. E. 'Unconfined fluid electrospun into high quality nanofibers from a plate edge.' *Polymer* 51 (2010): 4928–4936.
18. www.elmarco.com/electrospinning/electrospinning-technology/. Accessed 26 June 2017.
19. Molnar, K.; Nagy, Z. K. 'Corona-electrospinning: Needleless method for high-throughput continuous nanofiber production.' *Eur. Polym. J.* 74 (2016): 279–286.
20. Wu, H.; Zheng, Y.; Zeng, Y. 'A method for scale-up of co-electrospun nanofibers via flat core–shell structure spinneret.' *J. Appl. Polym. Sci.* 131 (2014): 41027.
21. Yan, X.; Marini, J.; Mulligan, R.; Deleault, A.; Sharma, U.; Brenner, M. P.; Rutledge, G. C.; Freyman, T.; Pham, Q. P. 'Slit-surface electrospinning: A novel process developed for high-throughput fabrication of core–sheath fibers.' *PLoS ONE* 10 (2015): e0125407.
22. Vysloužilová, L.; Buzgo, M.; Pokorny, P.; Chvojka, J.; Mickova, A.; Rampichova, M.; Kula, J.; Pejchar, K.; Bilek, M.; Lukas, D.; Amler, E. 'Needleless coaxial electrospinning: A novel approach to mass production of coaxial nanofibers.' *Int. J. Pharm.* 516 (2017): 293–300.
23. Jordahl, J. H.; Ramcharan, S.; Gregory, J. V.; Lahann, J. 'Needleless electrohydrodynamic cojetting of bicompartmental particles and fibers from an extended fluid interface.' *Macromol. Rapid Commun.* 38 (2017): 1600437.
24. Zhou, Z.; Wu, X.-F.; Ding, Y.; Yu, M.; Zhao, Y.; Jiang, L.; Xuan, C.; Sun, C. 'Needleless emulsion electrospinning for scalable fabrication of core–shell nanofibers.' *J. Appl. Polym. Sci.* 131 (2014): 40896.
25. Wang, Q.; Curtis, C. K.; Thoppey, N. M.; Bochinski, J. R.; Gorga, R. E.; Clarke, L. I. 'Unconfined, melt edge electrospinning from multiple, spontaneous, self-organized polymer jets.' *Mater. Res. Exp.* 1 (2014): 045304.
26. Lawson, C.; Stanishevsky, A.; Sivan, M.; Pokorny, P.; Lukáš, D. 'Rapid fabrication of poly(ε-caprolactone) nanofibers using needleless alternating current electrospinning.' *J. Appl. Polym. Sci.* 133 (2016): 43232.
27. Qi, S.; Craig, D. 'Recent developments in micro- and nanofabrication techniques for the preparation of amorphous pharmaceutical dosage forms.' *Adv. Drug Deliv. Rev.* 100 (2016): 67–84.
28. Wang, S.; Yang, Y.; Zhang, Y.; Fei, X.; Zhou, C.; Zhang, Y.; Li, Y.; Yang, Q.; Song, Y. 'Fabrication of large-scale superhydrophobic composite films with enhanced tensile properties by multinozzle conveyor belt electrospinning.' *J. Appl. Polym. Sci.* 131 (2014): 39735.
29. Krogstad, E. A.; Woodrow, K. A. 'Manufacturing scale-up of electrospun poly(vinyl alcohol) fibers containing tenofovir for vaginal drug delivery.' *Int. J. Pharm.* 475 (2014): 282–291.
30. Nagy, Z. K.; Balogh, A.; Demuth, B.; Pataki, H.; Vigh, T.; Szabo, B.; Molnar, K.; Schmidt, B. T.; Horak, P.; Marosi, G.; Verreck, G.; Van Assche, I.;

Brewster, M. E. 'High speed electrospinning for scaled-up production of amorphous solid dispersion of itraconazole.' *Int. J. Pharm.* 480 (2015): 137–142.

31. Demuth, B.; Farkas, A.; Balogh, A.; Bartosiewicz, K.; Kallai-Szabo, B.; Bertels, J.; Vigh, T.; Mensch, J.; Verreck, G.; Van Assche, I.; Marosi, G.; Nagy, Z. K. 'Lubricant-induced crystallization of itraconazole from tablets made of electrospun amorphous solid dispersion.' *J. Pharm. Sci.* 105 (2016): 2982–2988.
32. Demuth, B.; Farkas, A.; Pataki, H.; Balogh, A.; Szabo, B.; Borbas, E.; Soti, P. L.; Vigh, T.; Kiserdei, E.; Farkas, B.; Mensch, J.; Verreck, G.; Van Assche, I.; Marosi, G.; Nagy, Z. K. 'Detailed stability investigation of amorphous solid dispersions prepared by single-needle and high speed electrospinning.' *Int. J. Pharm.* 498 (2016): 234–244.
33. Wagner, I.; Nagy, Z. K.; Vass, P.; Fehér, C.; Barta, Z.; Vigh, T.; Sóti, P. L.; Harasztos, A. H.; Pataki, H.; Balogh, A.; Verreck, G.; Assche, I. V.; Marosi, G. 'Stable formulation of protein-type drug in electrospun polymeric fiber followed by tableting and scaling-up experiments.' *Polym. Adv. Technol.* 26 (2015): 1461–1467.
34. www.ich.org/home.html. Accessed 16 November 2017.
35. (a) https://ec.europa.eu/health/documents/eudralex/vol-4_en. Accessed 16 November 2017; (b) www.pharmpress.com/product/9780857112910/orangeguide. Accessed 16 November 2017.
36. www.imetechnologies.com/. Accessed 26 June 2017.
37. Alamein, M. A.; Liu, Q.; Stephens, S.; Skabo, S.; Warnke, F.; Bourke, R.; Heiner, P.; Warnke, P. H. 'Nanospiderwebs: Artificial 3D extracellular matrix from nanofibers by novel clinical grade electrospinning for stem cell delivery.' *Adv. Healthcare Mater.* 2 (2013): 702–717.
38. www.electrospinning.co.uk/. Accessed 26 June 2017.

8

Conclusions and Outlook

In this volume, we have explored in detail the use of polymer nanofibres in drug delivery. The majority of attention was paid to electrospinning, since this is the route which has received by far the most research attention for fabricating drug-loaded fibres. The different electrospinning techniques have been introduced, and guidance provided on how to begin a new experimental process. The products formed are related to the type of electrospinning undertaken, and we have seen that monoaxial spinning of a polymer solution yields monolithic fibres, while emulsion or coaxial spinning tends to result in core/shell structures. Three-liquid electrospinning can be used to prepare fibres with three layers, and side-by-side spinning to produce Janus fibres with two separate sides.

The types of drug delivery system that can be prepared with each electrospinning approach were described in detail, with a survey of examples from the literature presented to illustrate key points. In terms of monolithic fibres, a suitable choice of polymer can lead to fast-dissolving drug delivery systems (with a water-soluble hydrophilic polymer), extended release over hours or days (with insoluble or slowly degrading polymers) and targeted release (pH-sensitive polymers). Thermoresponsive systems can also be generated.

The monoaxial approach is advantageous because of its simplicity, but the high surface area of the fibres often causes an uncontrollable initial burst of release. This is a particular problem with high drug loadings. Electrospinning using suspensions or emulsions can help to ameliorate this issue. Emulsion spinning can also help to stabilise biomolecules such as proteins during the electrospinning process. Alternatively, a range of possibilities for making multilayer systems exist and can be used to provide more sophisticated release patterns. As well as their use in drug delivery, monolithic fibres can be employed as sacrificial templates for the self-assembly of higher-order objects.

Coaxial electrospinning offers the potential to solve a number of the problems of monoaxial spinning. For instance, making a core/shell fibre with the drug payload localised in the core can prevent burst release, although the formulation has to be carefully designed to do this successfully. Other release profiles which can be provided through coaxial spinning include biphasic release (with two phases occurring at different rates) and pH-sensitive release, targeting delivery to the small intestine. Multiple components can be included in the different compartments of the fibre and freed at different times. Since only one of the two solutions used for spinning need be electrospinnable, the coaxial approach can provide protection to protein drugs by incorporating them into the core of the fibres, with a protein-friendly aqueous solvent used for the core liquid. Alternatively, a pure solvent or solution of small molecules can be employed as the outer liquid; this yields monolithic fibres, but can help to prevent blocking of the spinneret or provide surface functionality. Triaxial electrospinning offers opportunities to provide even more complex products, but this comes at the cost of a more challenging fabrication process.

Janus fibres are difficult to prepare, because the two working liquids have a tendency to separate upon exiting the spinneret. They have thus received far less attention than monolithic or core/shell fibres. There are some approaches which can be taken to solve this problem, and several novel experimental methods have been reported in recent years, but at the time of writing we could find only a few reports of Janus drug delivery systems fabricated by electrospinning.

In addition to standard electrospinning performed with direct current (DC), a range of other methods to produce fibres exist. Alternating current (AC) electrospinning can be higher-throughput than the DC approach, and although it can be more difficult to obtain good-quality fibres, the functional performance of materials prepared by AC and DC spinning is very similar. Polymer melts can also be electrospun, producing fibres with diameters usually on the micron scale. This method avoids the use of any organic solvent, and thus the concomitant hazards associated with these, but it does require heat, which can lead to drug degradation.

Other approaches to fibre production use different sources of energy for solvent evaporation. Polymer-based fibres made by centrifugal spinning (where centrifugal force is used to evaporate solvent), solution blowing (exploiting a pressurised gas) and pressurised gyration (using both together) have all been explored for drug delivery, with promising results. Electrospinning can also be combined with blow spinning to produce drug-loaded fibres. These techniques are typically higher-throughput than standard lab electrospinning

Electrospinning has a sister technology, electrospraying, which uses the same principles but produces polymer-based particles. These also have an important role to play in drug delivery. Electrospraying and electrospinning can be combined to produce multi-functional materials.

Although electrospun fibres, and those prepared using the other techniques mentioned, have tremendous potential in drug delivery, the vast majority of studies to date have been undertaken on the lab scale. In the last few years, a number of technologies have emerged which permit the process to be scaled up to an industrial scale, and initial experiments using these have been very promising. However, more work is needed to explore scale-up and how the fibres prepared on the large scale compare with those made in the lab. The reproducibility of the materials prepared in different locations will need to be carefully established. There thus remains much work to be done before polymer fibre-based drug delivery systems can reach their full potential in improving human health and well-being.

Permissions

All chapters in this book were first published in ATFTPLPD, by Springer Nature; hereby published with permission under the Creative Commons Attribution License or equivalent. Every chapter published in this book has been scrutinized by our experts. Their significance has been extensively debated. The topics covered herein carry significant findings which will fuel the growth of the discipline. They may even be implemented as practical applications or may be referred to as a beginning point for another development.

The contributors of this book come from diverse backgrounds, making this book a truly international effort. This book will bring forth new frontiers with its revolutionizing research information and detailed analysis of the nascent developments around the world.

We would like to thank all the contributing authors for lending their expertise to make the book truly unique. They have played a crucial role in the development of this book. Without their invaluable contributions this book wouldn't have been possible. They have made vital efforts to compile up to date information on the varied aspects of this subject to make this book a valuable addition to the collection of many professionals and students.

This book was conceptualized with the vision of imparting up-to-date information and advanced data in this field. To ensure the same, a matchless editorial board was set up. Every individual on the board went through rigorous rounds of assessment to prove their worth. After which they invested a large part of their time researching and compiling the most relevant data for our readers.

The editorial board has been involved in producing this book since its inception. They have spent rigorous hours researching and exploring the diverse topics which have resulted in the successful publishing of this book. They have passed on their knowledge of decades through this book. To expedite this challenging task, the publisher supported the team at every step. A small team of assistant editors was also appointed to further simplify the editing procedure and attain best results for the readers.

Apart from the editorial board, the designing team has also invested a significant amount of their time in understanding the subject and creating the most relevant covers. They scrutinized every image to scout for the most suitable representation of the subject and create an appropriate cover for the book.

The publishing team has been an ardent support to the editorial, designing and production team. Their endless efforts to recruit the best for this project, has resulted in the accomplishment of this book. They are a veteran in the field of academics and their pool of knowledge is as vast as their experience in printing. Their expertise and guidance has proved useful at every step. Their uncompromising quality standards have made this book an exceptional effort. Their encouragement from time to time has been an inspiration for everyone.

The publisher and the editorial board hope that this book will prove to be a valuable piece of knowledge for researchers, students, practitioners and scholars across the globe.

Index

www.ingramcontent.com/pod-product-compliance
Lightning Source LLC
LaVergne TN
LVHW051044220926
848485LV00001BA/9
* 9 7 8 1 6 3 9 2 7 5 5 4 0 *